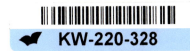

Contents

PERGAMON INTERNATIONAL LIBRARY
of Science, Technology, Engineering and Social Studies
The 1000-volume original paperback library in aid of education,
industrial training and the enjoyment of leisure
Publisher: Robert Maxwell, M.C.

6.00

J. L. Jones.
Bristol Dental
Hospital. Sept '81

ORAL DIAGNOSIS

Other titles of interest:

BROTHWELL: Dental Anthropology

DAVIS & BOLIN: Symptom Analysis and Physical Diagnosis in Medicine

ELDER & NEILL: Biomedical Technology in Hospital Diagnosis

EMMELIN & ZOTTERMAN: Oral Physiology

JAMES *et al:* Advances in Fluorine and Dental Caries Prevention, Volume 4

SCHMIDT & KEIL: Polarizing Microscopy of Dental Tissues

ORAL DIAGNOSIS

A Handbook of Modern Diagnostic Techniques
Used to Investigate
Clinical Problems in Dentistry

BY

W. R. TYLDESLEY

D.D.S., Ph.D., F.D.S.R.C.S.
Reader in Dental Surgery, University of Liverpool

SECOND EDITION

PERGAMON PRESS

OXFORD · NEW YORK · TORONTO · SYDNEY · PARIS · FRANKFURT

U.K.	Pergamon Press Ltd., Headington Hill Hall, Oxford OX3 0BW, England
U.S.A.	Pergamon Press Inc., Maxwell House, Fairview Park, Elmsford, New York 10523, U.S.A.
CANADA	Pergamon of Canada Ltd., 75 The East Mall, Toronto, Ontario, Canada
AUSTRALIA	Pergamon Press (Aust.) Pty. Ltd., 19a Boundary Street, Rushcutters Bay, N.S.W. 2011, Australia
FRANCE	Pergamon Press SARL, 24 rue des Ecoles, 75240 Paris, Cedex 05, France
FEDERAL REPUBLIC OF GERMANY	Pergamon Press GmbH, 6242 Kronberg-Taunus, Pferdstrasse 1, Federal Republic of Germany

First edition 1969

Second edition 1978

British Library Cataloguing in Publication Data

Tyldesley, William Randolph
Oral diagnosis. - 2nd ed.
1. Teeth - Diseases - Diagnosis
I. Title
617.6'07'5   RK308   78-40385
ISBN 0-08-021543-2 Hardcover
ISBN 0-08-023181-0 Flexicover

In order to make this volume available as economically and as rapidly as possible the author's typescript has been reproduced in its original form. This method unfortunately has its typographical limitations but it is hoped that they in no way distract the reader.

Printed in Great Britain by William Clowes and Sons Ltd, Beccles.

Preface

The first edition of this book was written in an attempt to help the dental student by bringing together descriptions of the diagnostic techniques used to investigate clinical problems in dentistry. In the intervening ten years there have been radical changes in the scope of the investigations which are regularly carried out on patients in the care of dental surgeons. These particularly reflect the great widening of interest in the relationship between systemic disease and changes in the oral cavity. It is hoped that the present book will provide a convenient source of reference for students faced with this ever expanding field and that it will provide a suitable background for the understanding of the procedures described.

No attempt has been made to illustrate all the clinical conditions mentioned or to provide pathological detail. Textbooks and atlases of oral medicine, radiography, histopathology and so on will provide this kind of information. The most profusely illustrated chapter is that concerning lesions of the teeth. This subject, of obvious major importance to most dentists, depends largely on visual recognition of the conditions and it was felt justified to include a wider range of illustration than in the other chapters. Elsewhere the emphasis has been placed predominantly on methods of investigation rather than on the illustration of lesions.

No short book dealing with so wide a subject can be absolutely comprehensive, but it is hoped that the basic diagnostic techniques have been indicated for most of the conditions likely to arise in either the general or hospital practice of dentistry.

Acknowledgements

Material has been generously made available by the following:- Mr. P.D. Bird, Dr. J. Bradley, Coulter Electronics Limited, Professor K. McCarthy, Dr. N.R. Rowell and Mr. F. Taylor-Monks.

Permission to reprint figures has been kindly given by the editors of the British Dental Journal, the British Journal of Oral Surgery and The Practitioner.

The arduous task of preparing the script for publication has been carried out by Miss Linda Byron.

Chapter I

Examination of the Patient

The first step in the investigation of any patient should be a review of all available notes, correspondence and other similar documents. This background information is best acquired before the patient is actually seen, the lead given being valuable in planning the approach to the patient as well as being essential for the subsequent diagnosis.

When the examination of the patient is being carried out, all significant facts should at once be added to the records. The necessity of making full notes at the time of examination cannot be overstressed. Memory for details of one patient amongst many may be very short and it is essential that full information should be available to any subsequent colleague who may attend the patient. Quite apart from the invaluable nature of full notes from a dental or medical viewpoint, their importance in any matter involving legal proceedings is clear.

It is a personal view that complex charts for the recording of results of an oral examination are unnecessary and that relevant facts are better recorded in words, rather than as a mark against a previously determined entry in a diagnostic chart. The value of such aids, however, is that there is a clearly laid down routine which must be followed in every case. Without a set chart it is important that a routine form of procedure should be adopted and adhered to for the examination of all patients. With an established routine, the likelihood of significant omissions grows less and the task of recording the examination is simplified.

The precise order of the examination may be subject to individual variation depending on the circumstances - for instance, it may be considered more appropriate for the extra-oral examination to be carried out before that of the intra-oral structures. The comprehensive scheme of procedure as described is perhaps less well suited to the circumstances of general dental practice as to a specialist clinic in the hospital environment and some degree of 'short-circuiting' of the full examination procedure may be considered inevitable. However, if such a contraction is carried out then it must be with a full awareness of omissions.

The first phase of the examination occurs as the patient enters the room and during any conversation preliminary to the case-history taking. It is not suggested that the dentist should act as a "spot diagnostician" of medical or psychiatric complaints, but the recognition of sick, frightened or mentally disturbed patients may help greatly in determining the line of

1

investigation. The powers of observation which enable the expert diagnostician to recognize these factors may be aided to a certain degree by personal flair, and to a great extent by experience, but are based firmly on a sound knowledge of the relevant pathology.

The history taking should begin with the personal details of the patient's name, address, age, marital status and occupation, if these have not been already entered in the notes. If they have been previously obtained, these details should be read before the examination proceeds. The outlook of varying types of patient differs vastly in relation to such matters as aesthetics, degree of reaction to pain, tolerance of discomfort and so on, and it is well worthwhile to have the patient's personal details in mind when attempting to assess certain conditions.

The patient should be asked first of all the nature of his complaint. It may well differ in a quite startling manner from the details given in previous notes or correspondence. This may be simply due to the different emphasis the patient may be expected to place on his symptoms, but may also imply a change in the condition or the onset of a secondary condition. The order in which symptoms have occurred should be carefully determined - often a much more difficult task than at first imagined.

It is worth spending a little time in sorting out the confused details of a history which may be told in reverse order - not unnaturally so, since more recent and possibly more urgent symptoms will be uppermost in the patient's mind.

Details of the relevant medical and dental histories should next be taken. So far as the medical details are concerned, it is often necessary to ask directly whether there have been past illnesses, whether the patient is at present receiving medical treatment and for what, and whether he is at present taking any drugs. Patients are often reluctant to volunteer information on what they may consider to be irrelevant past conditions and direct questioning must be used. The precise questions asked must evidently depend to some extent on the circumstances. Quite clearly a history of rheumatic fever, coronary disease or some similar condition is of high significance in all branches of dental practice and must always be uncovered. In order to assist the patient to reply fully a list of significant condit- ions may be prepared and shown before the examination. In Table 1 is shown the text of a printed card, initially produced for use in the Dental Hospital environment, which could be easily adapted for use in practice conditions. In the specialist clinic the inter-relation between oral and generalised diseases may be of greater than usual significance and the direct questioning must evidently be taken further.

TABLE 1

PLEASE READ THIS AND GIVE IT TO
THE REGISTRAR

Have you had any of the
following conditions?

1. Heart Disease
2. Lung Disease
3. Rheumatic Fever
4. High Blood Pressure
5. Kidney Disease
6. Diabetes, Hyperthyroidism,
   Porphyria
7. Blood Disease, Anaemia,
   Excessive Haemorrhage
8. Epilepsy, Fainting Attacks
9. Nervous Trouble
10. Hepatitis

Are you

1. Allergic to Anything?
2. On any Medicine or Drugs?
3. Pregnant?

The significance of the questions regarding the taking of
drugs is obvious in view of the increasing numbers of patients
maintained on long-term therapies. Many modern therapeutic
regimes produce side reactions which affect the oral cavity. For
instance a wide range of drugs, including anti-depressants and
anti-hypertensives, produce xerostomia - dry mouth - as a side
effect. Other examples are the production of a sore tongue
during treatment by wide spectrum antibiotics and the precipitation of thrush (acute pseudo-membranous candidiasis) by the use
of systemic cortico-steroids. There are many other similar
examples. Often the patient is quite unaware of the connection
between the drug therapy and the side effects and again direct
questionning must be used.

When developmental anomalies are present or suspected, as in
the case of anodontia, defects of tooth structure, facial dystro-
phies and so on, the family history takes on considerable importance. The family photograph album may be of great use in
detecting the degree of involvement of other members of the
family, including those deceased. In the same way, a series of
photographs, however simple or technically faulty, can be
assembled by most patients in order to show their facial characteristics over the years, and these may prove very useful in the
assessment of slowly increasing facial deformity.

In the giving of a dental history, the patient may often find
great difficulty in placing chronologically the treatment that
has been carried out and considerable patience is often needed to
assemble facts in the correct order. Although the patient's

description of past treatment may appear somewhat exaggerated,
it is rarely advisable to dismiss too lightly stories of difficult extractions, post-operative haemorrhage and similar
incidents which may be all too easily repeated in the most
inconvenient circumstances.

The examination. After taking the history the examination of
the mouth may be carried out, taking in order teeth, soft
tissues, bone structures and extraoral structures. It is advisable to maintain a routine procedure for all cases and to
examine, for example, the teeth in a fixed order, say from left
to right in the mandibular teeth, followed by the same order in
the maxillary teeth. If a routine of this nature is not
maintained, then omissions may occur.

When examining the patient, a comfortable position for both
patient and operator is a help in reducing strains, both physical
and mental. Adequate illumination is absolutely essential, and
it is a great help if the light can be focused on the mouth
alone when that is required; many patients are apprehensive when
undergoing examination and a dazzling light in the eyes does
much to increase the patient's discomfort. Similarly the
adoption of an easy chair-side manner and the use of a vocab-
ulary adapted to the patient's comprehension will be repaid with
increased relaxation of the patient, and a consequently better
history. If patients are to be examined away from the properly
equipped dental surgery - for instance in a hospital bed - the
use of some form of portable illumination is essential for
successful intra-oral examination. The use of ambient room
light in this situation may lead to gross errors of omission.
Not only the intensity but also the colour of the light may
affect the accuracy of the examination - some mucosal lesions
may become virtually invisible when viewed in the illumination
provided by certain tinted dental lamps.

The teeth. The teeth must first be charted, those absent
being noted. It must be remembered that teeth missing from the
arch may be unerupted, congenitally absent or have been
extracted and it is often quite impossible to differentiate
between these possibilities without radiographic evidence. Each
tooth must be systematically viewed and explored on all surfaces
by means of sharp probes for the presence of caries. To aid in
the visual examination the teeth should be dry and, if there is
much saliva, drying either by an air syringe or with cotton wool
is essential for a satisfactory view. The probes used must be
sharp and usually a sickle type and a double ended Briault type
probe are all that are necessary.

As each tooth is viewed any colour change is noted, together
with any evidence of hypoplasia, erosion, attrition or abrasion.
Testing for sensitivity to percussion is carried out gently with
the reversed end of a mirror handle. If the vitality of any
tooth is suspect, then pulp testing should be carried out. The
methods adopted and the significance of their results are discussed in Chapter V.

Occlusion. The teeth, having been viewed individually, must
next be examined as a functional whole, malocclusions of all
kinds being recorded. If treatment of malocclusion or traumatic
occlusion is contemplated, then study impressions of the initial
state are essential to aid in a considered diagnosis.

Periodontal structures. These should next be investigated.
The presence of supra- or subgingival calculus is noted, the
latter by passing a probe gently and atraumatically to the depth
of the gingival crevice. The presence of materia alba and the
state of oral hygiene is also noted. The gingival soft tissues
are carefully visualized, noting any change of contour, colour
or surface texture. Any recession of the gingival margin, and
consequent exposure of cementum, is noted, and loss of attachment
of the teeth estimated by gently testing for mobility. Where
minimal changes in a tooth are suspected, the test for mobility
is best done by placing the finger over the buccal surface of
the tooth and the adjacent teeth and allowing the patient to
come into occlusion. Small movements are then easily detected
by the examining finger. More gross forms of mobility are tested
for by gently applying pressure to the suspect tooth in a linguo-
buccal direction. Instruments should be used for this, not
fingers, which hide the tooth and themselves deform and may
convey inaccurate sensations of movement. Any exudate from the
gingival margin after gentle pressure must also be noted.

The oral mucosa. The whole surface of the oral mucosa must
be visualized and examined for any abnormality. In order to
retract the lips and cheeks sufficiently to expose fully the
sulci, a dental mirror used as a retractor is invaluable. For
examination of the tongue, it should be held between fingers and
thumb using a gauze napkin and traction gently applied both
forward and laterally; in this way the best view of the lateral
margin of the tongue and the floor of the mouth is given. The
anterior part of the floor of the mouth is then visualised,
together with the ventral surface of the tongue, by asking the
patient to touch the palate with the tongue. The tonsillar
areas and posterior pharyngeal wall are examined by asking the
patient to say 'Ah' whilst gently pressing the dorsum of the
tongue with the dental mirror. For a brief period the soft
palate is elevated and the view is clear. For this view the
light should be adjusted to be directed horizontally from behind
the examiner's head (in these circumstances the Ear, Nose &
Throat surgeon would use a head mirror).

Palpation is used to assess the texture of any lesion and to
detect induration. Swellings in the substance of the soft
tissues are best examined by bimanual palpation, the examining
fingers lying on each side of the tissue mass. Palpation of
structures within the floor of the mouth is made easier by a
gentle upward pressure in the submandibular area by which the
tissues are lifted and well defined.

Fluid filled lesions in the soft tissues are detected by
observing the "fluid thrill" passed through the lesion between

examining fingers placed on each side of it. It may be difficult
to differentiate between a deeply seated fluid filled lesion and
a very soft solid tissue mass. Aspiration biopsy (Chapter III)
will assist the diagnosis in these cases.

   The facial skeleton.   The facial contours are viewed from the
front. Any asymmetry is noted, remembering that virtually all
faces are to some extent asymmetrical. Swellings may be confirmed by gentle palpation of the facial skeleton, always palpating bilaterally to compare with the unaffected side. If a
swelling of the upper third of the face is noted it is better
seen by viewing downmwards from over the head of the patient.

   Intraorally the skeleton may again be palpated bilaterally,
the fingers passing lingually and buccally over the mucosa
covering the mandible, and up the ascending ramus. In the maxilla the exploring finger passes buccally and palatally over the
alveolar process and should be carried posteriorly to palpate
the tuberosities distal to any standing teeth.

   Gentle pressure should be brought to bear on any swelling
found. Its texture, sensitivity and tendency to spring or
produce the crackling characteristic of thin plates of bone,
should be noted.

   The temporomandibular joints.   The temporomandibular joint is
palpated by a single finger placed slightly anterior and below
the external auditory meatus, whilst standing in front of the
patient. When maintaining this position, the patient is asked to
open and close the mouth and to perform protrusive and lateral
movements. Undue movements of the condyle head and clicking of
the joint can be felt quite plainly, whilst in cases of joint
dysfunction, the patient may complain of pain on the slightest
pressure from the palpating finger when the mouth is opened.
Further joint sounds are well heard by the use of a stethoscope
placed over the condyle head.

   Standing centrally in front of the patient, any deviation in
opening and closing the mouth may be noted, together with any
abnormal cuspal guidance. It is often in the last few millimetres of closure that some abnormal lateral movement occurs,
and this must be carefully looked for. The examination of the
temporomandibular joint and its associated structures and the
significance of various signs associated with abnormal joint
function are further discussed in Chapter VIII.

   The neck.   Finally, the soft tissues of the face and neck
must be palpated and for this the best position is behind the
patient. Bilateral palpation of the face, parotid and submandibular salivary glands and neck is carried out, followed by
careful search for prominent lymph nodes in the neck. For this
examination the patient must relax the neck muscles by bending
the head slightly forwards and to the respective side whilst the
regions of the submandibular, submental, auricular and cervical
nodes are palpated on each side in turn.

Other associated structures. Examination of the eyes, skin,
ears and sinuses must of necessity be confined to a simple
inspection. Further clinical examination is best left to a
colleague in the appropriate specialty, as is the treatment of
most conditions not specifically oral or dental in nature. In a
hospital environment examination of the extra-oral structures may
well be carried further by the specialist dental surgeon who will
have been trained in the use of the appropriate techniques. The
illuminated auriscope, for instance, may be of value in examining
not only the external auditory meatus and eardrum, but also the
anterior nasal structures. A knowledge of the clinical features
of skin diseases may also be of great value to the dental
diagnostition - many diseases of the skin present with oral
lesions and it is evidently important that the dentist dealing
with the oral lesions should have some acquaintance with the
wider aspects of the conditions involved. This does not necessarily imply however that the dental surgeon is the person best
qualified to deal with the subsequent treatment. Indeed the
greatest value of a careful examination of the extra-oral structures may well be the opportunity for prompt reference of the
patient to the appropriate specialist.

Diagnostic Terminology
    Following the general examination of the patient a provisional
diagnosis may be reached. If the situation is an uncomplicated
one a definitive diagnosis may be achieved at this stage but in
other circumstances the results of special investigations may
have to be considered before a firm conclusion may be reached.
If a number of possibilities need to be considered equally a
differential diagnosis must be made and the various possibilities
explored before reaching a final decision. Similarly a tentative
diagnosis, made on relatively thin evidence, must be substant-
iated by a fuller study.

Special Investigations
    The subsequent chapters are devoted largely to details of
special investigations - both the clinical investigation of
individual lesions or abnormal structures and the application of
laboratory tests. These special investigations follow the
general examination and are dictated by the initial findings.
The extent to which the special investigations should be carried
out depends greatly on the circumstances of the case. Many of
the laboratory tests described are time consuming as well as
expensive to perform and patients should be carefully selected
before any scheme of detailed investigation is embarked upon.

Radiography
    The special investigation most commonly carried out in dentist-
ry is the taking of radiographs. Although the indiscriminate use
of these is obviously to be deprecated, the risk of radiation
damage from dental radiography is absolutely minimal (with the
adoption of simple safety precautions), and there is rarely any
excuse for not obtaining them if they are necessary for diagnosis.

    Even in relatively routine diagnostic problems there is every-

thing to be gained by obtaining adequate well positioned radiographs. For a complete assessment of the dental condition full
mouth periapical films, properly positioned to include the apices
of the teeth, are mandatory. As a simple screening test for
gross pathology, however, the panoramic equipment now generally
available which produces views of the mandible and the maxilla
together with the associated structures on a single film is quite
invaluable. The use of radiographs in the diagnosis of caries is
discussed in Chapter V.

The dental surgeon being for the most part his own diagnostic
radiologist, care must always be taken in the recognition of
anatomical landmarks which may be mistaken for pathological
conditions; the antrum and the mental or incisive foramen being
foremost amongst the readily mistaken structures (Figs. 1.1.).
Similarly, the superimposition of structures must always be kept
in mind and, if necessary, any possible errors obviated by the
taking of additional films differently angulated.

The use of contrast media may, occasionally, be valuable in
the demonstration of patent ducts or sinuses or to demark clearly
a vague osteolytic lesion. In a very few instances angiographic
techniques (predominantly carotid arteriography) may be applied
to delineate a vascular neoplasm or other similar abnormality
(Figs. 1.2, 1.3 and 1.4). Such methods, of course, are entirely
the province of the specialist radiologist. The major use of
contrast media in oral diagnosis, however, is in the injection
of the salivary ducts to produce sialographs, and to gain
information regarding the condition of the salivary glands. The
technique of this is described in Chapter IX. Other specialized
radiographic techniques are occasionally used in oral diagnostic
procedures and these also are referred to in subsequent chapters.
Diagnostic methods rarely applied to the oral tissues are also
subsequently referred to in the appropriate chapters -
thermography, ultrasound and radioisotope tracing are among these
infrequently used but occasionally valuable modern techniques.

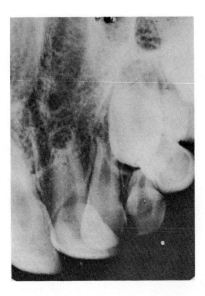

Fig. 1.1. Superimposed incisive foramen resembling an apical lesion. An unusually wide foramen may be mistaken for a midline cyst on radiographs.

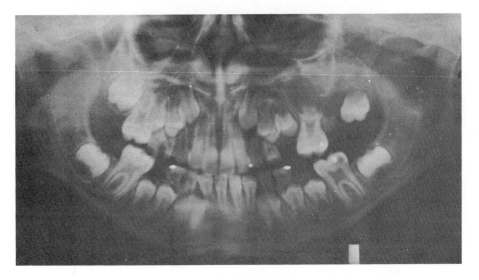

Fig. 1.2. Panoramic radiograph showing osteolytic lesion in the left maxilla, suspected of being a haemangioma. Contrast radiography was used to help confirm this diagnosis (Figs. 1.3, 1.4).

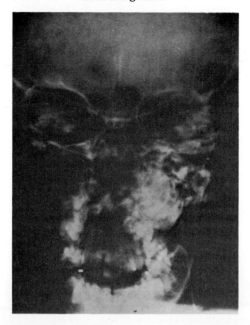

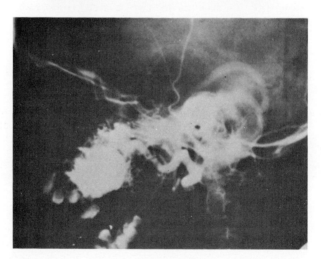

Fig. 1.3 and 1.4. Carotid angiograms confirming blood flow in the lesion shown in Fig. 1.2. Films taken during injection of radiopaque fluid into the left carotid artery.

Chapter II

Laboratory Investigations

The clinical and radiographic examination of the patient
having been completed, it must be decided whether further investigations are needed. These may be either to confirm a suspected
disorder, or obtain more information before the diagnosis is
provisionally made. Many of these investigations require
laboratory facilities and some of these are described below.
There are many other haematological and biochemical tests which
might occasionally be needed in the diagnosis of oral conditions
and, in particular, of diseases of the oral mucosa. The ones
specified here are, however, generally adequate for a full
investigation of the majority of the conditions which are likely
to be encountered in dentistry.

S.I. units (Systéme International) were introduced in 1960 and
subsequently adopted in many countries as biological units based
on fundamental measurements such as the metre and the kilogram.
Not all organizations are convinced of the superiority of this
system and, indeed, some units are so unwieldy as to be unadopted
by any groups of workers. Perhaps the most significant change in
the reporting of biochemical data is the use of the mole (or
fractions of the mole) as a unit of concentration. In using this
particular convention the reporting implies a function of molecular activity, rather than of simple mass. An example of an S.I.
unit which has not been adopted is the pascal as a measurement of
blood pressure - the present convention of "mm of mercury" is so
well established that it has been generally accepted that any
attempted change would lead to misunderstandings. In this chapter
units are expressed both conventionally and in S.I. units. The
S.I. units are added in brackets to the conventional figures (See
also Table IV).

Blood

Examination of a sample of the patient's blood is valuable in
three situations; as a screening procedure to aid the diagnosis
of an unknown condition; to help confirm a tentative diagnosis;
and to investigate a suspected disorder of the blood clotting
mechanism. It has become accepted that a variety of oral lesions
may occur in patients suffering from abnormalities of the blood -
particularly those with anaemias, latent anaemias and similar
conditions. It has also been shown that such lesions are non-
specific and that they may occur in the very early stages of the
disease. In such cases, therefore, it is necessary to carry out
a careful investigation of the haematological status of the
patients and to extend the tests well beyond those used in simple
screening procedures.

Collection
     For most tests, blood is taken either from a vein or from
capillaries. To obtain venous blood, the patient should be
seated or lying (fairly frequently a patient faints, although a
well-performed venepuncture is quite painless). A tourniquet is
placed firmly round the upper arm, or, if assistance is available,
the upper arm can be tightly encircled and gripped by two hands.
The skin over the cubital fossa is cleaned with alcohol and the
skin and vein are punctured by the collecting needle (about 21
gauge) used with the bevel upwards, attached to a sterile syringe
of about 10 to 25 ml capacity. After aspiration shows a small
amount of blood indicating that the needle is in the vein, the
tourniquet is released, a few seconds allowed for the establish-
ment of normal flow and the required amount of blood collected.
The needle is then withdrawn and pressure is applied to the
puncture with a sterile swab for a few moments to prevent further
bleeding. A small dressing may be used to cover the puncture
site for a day or so, although this is not strictly necessary.

     For most examinations not involving the clotting properties of
the blood, it should be emptied from the collecting syringe into
bottles containing an anticoagulant. This may be heparin, added
at a concentration of 0.5 mg per 5 ml of blood, although a more
commonly used anticoagulant is a mixture of ammonium oxalate and
potassium oxalate. It is obvious that blood so treated cannot be
used for the estimation of nitrogen or of potassium and, in these
cases, a single oxalate salt is used. Ready prepared disposable
plastic bottles are now widely available containing the proper
amount and type of anticoagulants suitable for different purposes.

     Small amounts of capillary blood, which are required for many
tests, may be obtained by puncturing the lobe of the ear or the
finger to a depth of 2 mm or so with a sharp lancet or needle.
There are many patterns of blood lancet available, some with
depth guards and some with a spring action. Needless to say,
whatever instrument is utilized must, like all equipment used on
patients for blood collection, be adequately sterilized; sterile
disposable lancets of simple design are now most widely used.
The first drop or two of blood should be discarded, and only the
further drops used in the examination. The puncture should not
be squeezed as this may express tissue serum and dilute the
blood. No further action is necessary to protect the puncture
when bleeding has stopped, which it normally does in a very short
time.

Automatic Blood Examination Systems
     Until relatively recently the usual method of examination of a
blood specimen in the laboratory has been carried out by simple
means. For example, direct visual counting of the red cells may
be carried out by diluting the blood with an isotonic solution,
filling a counting chamber of known depth with the diluted blood
and then counting, under a microscope, the number of red cells
seen over a known area ruled out on the base of the counting
chamber. It is then a matter of simple arithmetic to calculate
the number of cells present in a given volume of original blood.

The white cells may be counted in a similar manner, either at the
same time as the red cell count or following lysis of the red
cells in order to leave the white cells exposed.

In recent years, however, such laborious and relatively inaccurate methods have been increasingly replaced by the use of
automated systems in which virtually all the normally required
haematological values may be accurately and automatically
obtained. The particle counting is carried out by passing the
diluted blood through a narrow aperture or through a narrow
chamber. The count is then accomplished either by measuring
electrical field changes in the area of the aperture, by
measuring fluctuations in light reflected from the particles or
by some similar method. In the use of these systems it is
necessary only to supply a single sample of blood and, with the
more complete apparatus, the various indices are printed out
automatically within a very short time of the sample being fed
to the machine (Fig. 2.1.). Not only are these systems fast but
they are also accurate and by their use such measurements as the
erythrocyte count, previously considered to be an inaccurate
measure, may now be considered to be an accurate and comparable
figure.

Not all laboratories have such equipment; the expense is
considerable and there are still many small hospital laboratories
in which such automation has not been introduced. However, with
centralization of facilities it seems highly likely that in the
very near future non-automated forms of haematological study will
be considered completely out of date.

Routine Blood Examination
    For the routine screening procedure as an aid to diagnosis it
is usual to carry out only three examinations. These are a haemoglobin estimation, a cell count and a survey of a stained film
for abnormal cell forms. If any abnormality in these is found,
then further tests may be utilized. This simple screening
procedure is sufficient to give some indication of most fully
developed blood disorders and to indicate the lines of further
tests, but is inadequate to show up the early changes of anaemias
or of latent anaemias. As has been pointed out, oral changes may
provide the first clinical indication of the presence of these
conditions at a stage when haematological change is minimal. It
is, therefore, necessary to extend the blood examination in these
cases to include estimations of serum iron, total iron binding
capacity and saturation in order to detect latent anaemia. Serum
B_{12} and folate estimation must also be performed if there is any
possibility of an early megaloblastic anaemia, whilst an erythrocyte sedimentation rate estimation is a valuable but non-
specific indicator of basic pathological change. Deficiencies or
abnormalities of the clotting system will not be shown up by this
procedure, except occasionally by the presence of a secondary
anaemia.

Haemoglobin Estimation

The estimation of haemoglobin is not carried out by direct
chemical methods but by colour comparison with standards which
vary in the differing types of apparatus; all give reasonably
comparable results.

The results of haemoglobin estimation can be given in two
ways. The best and most accurate way is to express the result in
grammes of haemoglobin per 100 ml. In the S.I. system of units
100 ml is expressed as 1 decilitre (dl) and the haemoglobin
concentration is consequently expressed as g/dl. The second
method, still much employed, is to express the haemoglobin of the
blood under examination as a percentage of the "normal" value
taken as standard. The inaccuracy in this type of result lies in
the difficulty in defining a normal value, since this latter
varies with age and between the sexes. Frequently the haemoglobin
may be reported in both ways (e.g. Hb = 90 per cent = 13.3 g/100
ml).

Normal values for the adult male can be taken as varying from
14 to 18 g/100 ml and for the adult female 12 to 16 g/100 ml.
With mean values taken as 16 g/100 ml for males and 14 g/100 ml
for females this corresponds to an approximate percentage range
of from 85 to 115 per cent. At birth the haemoglobin concentration is high (of the order of 18 g/100 ml), but within a few
days this is reduced until at one year the expected value is
about 11g/100 ml. From this age the value gradually rises to the
full adult value at puberty. In old age the haemoglobin level is
found to fall and the normal values are a little lower than in
middle life.

Erythrocyte Count

In spite of the increased accuracy of erythrocyte counting
introduced by automatic methods the absolute value is still
considered as being relatively unimportant in diagnosis as compared to other indices.

Normal values for the red cell count may be taken as 4.5 to
6.5 million per mm^3 in adult males and 4 to 5.5 million per mm^3
in adult females. (S.I. units - x 10^{12}/1).

Packed cell volume   The packed cell volume of the erythrocytes
(P.C.V.) or haematrocrit value is obtained by centrifuging a
sample of the oxalated blood in a calibrated tube. The volume of
the sedimented cells is read directly from the calibrations on
the haematocrit tube, the volume of the white cells being
ignored as insignificant compared with that of the red cells.
The result is expressed as a percentage of the volume of the
blood sample. Normal values vary from 40 to 50 per cent in
males, from 35 to 45 per cent in females.

Mean corpuscular volume   The mean corpuscular volume or mean
cell volume (M.C.V.) is the average volume of the erythrocytes
and is directly calculated from the packed cell volume and the
erythrocyte count. The normal values vary from 76 to 96 μ^3.
(S.I. unit - fl).

Mean corpuscular haemoglobin.   The mean corpuscular haemoglobin (M.C.H.) represents the average weight of haemoglobin present in one erythrocyte. It is calculated from the red cell count and the haemoglobin estimation. The normal range is from 27 to 32 $\mu\mu$g. (S.I. unit - pg).

Mean corpuscular haemoglobin concentration.   The mean corpuscular haemoglobin concentration (M.C.H.C.) is a measure of the average concentration of haemoglobin in the erythrocytes. It can be directly calculated from the packed cell volume and the haemoglobin estimation. The normal values range from 32 to 36 g per cent.

The previous three values (M.C.V., M.C.H. and M.C.H.C.) are not normally obtained as part of an investigation for oral conditions. They are, however, used in the differential diagnosis of anaemias, which frequently first present with oral symptoms such as glossitis or stomatitis.

Colour index.   The colour index is sometimes used to express the concentration of haemoglobin in each red cell as a proportion of that in a normal cell. The use of this arbitrary value for the normal cell robs the figure of any absolute significance, although it is still used as a relative test, particularly in the diagnosis of anaemias.

The colour index is arrived at by assuming values of haemoglobin of about 15g/100 ml and an erythrocyte count of 5 million per mm^3. The haemoglobin concentration and erythrocyte count of the blood under test are calculated as percentages of these values. The colour index is then arrived at by dividing the percentage of haemoglobin by the percentage of erythrocytes. If the blood under test is "normal", then the percentages calculated will be 100 in both cases and the colour index will be 1.

It will be seen that, since the index includes two measured values expressed as rather arbitrary percentages, it cannot convey more information than the two values given separately. It has, however, proved a convenient term for clinicians and is still occasionally used. It is included here rather for completeness than to recommend its adoption as a routine diagnostic test - the mean corpuscular haemoglobin is a much more reliable test for the same factors.

White Cell Count
The number of white cells present in the blood of a normal individual varies from 5,000 to 10,000 per mm^3. (S.I. units - 5 to 10 x 10^9/1). There are variations in the count in the course of a day, the maximum being attained in the afternoon. The total white cell count is no more than a rough indication of some pathological process at work, the relative proportions of cell types present often being of much greater significance. However, as a screening procedure the total count is a satisfactory measure.

It should always be borne in mind, however, that in, for
example, a leukaemic condition the cell forms may be largely
abnormal whilst the total white count may still remain within
the accepted normal limits. For this reason a screening white
cell count should be routinely accompanied by a search of a
stained film for abnormal cell forms.

<u>Blood Film Examination</u>

In order to determine the normality or otherwise of the blood
cells it is necessary to study a stained film of the blood.
This is produced by spreading a small drop of blood evenly in a
thin film over almost the whole of a microscope slide by using
the edge of a second slide as a spreader. The film is air dried
and then may be stained by one of a number of available stains.
These are mostly complex polychrome substances containing methyl
alcohol which also acts as a fixative for the film. The best
known of these stains are Giemsa's, Leishmann's and Wright's.
After staining, the film is dried out and viewed directly, without a cover glass, under the oil immersion lens. With a successful technique the erythrocytes stain orange-pink, the nuclei
blue-purple and eosinophilic and basophilic granules in the
polymorphs stain red and blue respectively. Consistency in
staining technique is evidently important and this has been
recognised by the introduction of automatic staining machines
which operate under closely controlled conditions.

TABLE II

VARIATION IN SIZE AND SHAPE OF ERYTHROCYTES

Description	Erythrocyte characteristics	Seen in
Hypochromic	Pale staining	Iron deficiency anaemia
Hyperchromic	Dense staining	Pernicious anaemia
Microcytic	Small	Iron deficiency anaemia
Macrocytic	Large (10-12μ)	Pernicious anaemia
Megalocytic	Very large (12-25μ)	Pernicious anaemia
Anisocytosis	Much variation in size	Most anaemias
Poikilocytosis	Much variation in shape	Most anaemias
Spherocytic	Spherical	Congenital haemolytic anaemias
Target cell	Concentrically stained	Any chronic anaemia
Erythroblast	Nucleated	Denote excessive erythropoiesis
(i) Normoblast	Normal size	After haemorrhage, very severe anaemias and leukaemias
(ii) Microblast		
(iii) Megaloblast	Large size	Pernicious anaemia, carcinoma stomach, after total gastrectomy
Reticulocyte	Reticulated when stained with vital stains	If higher than 1 per cent in adults - an active marrow response to a demand for eryth-rocytes.

If it is wished to stain reticulocytes a technique known as vital staining is carried out by mixing the blood sample with an equal volume of cresyl blue solution before the preparation of the smear, which may then be stained in the normal manner. This is not a normal technique in routine blood examination and is carried out only when specifically requested.

In a stained film the erythrocytes may show variations in depths of staining, size, shape and maturity. The normal erythrocytes appear as single discs, slightly more intensely stained towards the edge with an average diameter 7.3μ. The meanings of some of the terms used to describe variations from the normal are given in Table II together with an indication of some of the conditions in which these forms may occur.

The relative proportions of the differing varieties of white cells (a differential count) are obtained by counting a large number of cells present in a stained film (250 for an approximate result, 1,000 for an accurate one), classifying them when counting. The cells should be taken from different areas of the film which ought to be reasonably evenly spread as shown by low power examination. Pathological varieties of cells are, of course, carefully noted in addition to counting the normal forms. The distribution of leukocytes in the blood of normal adults is shown in Table III.

TABLE III

AVERAGE DISTRIBUTION OF LEUKOCYTES
IN NORMAL ADULT BLOOD

	Percentage
Lymphocytes	25-30
Monocytes	2-6
Polymorphonuclear neutrophils	60-70
Eosinophils	1-4
Basophils	0-0.5

Total number of leukocytes in normal adult blood; 4,000-11,000 per mm^3. ($4-11 \times 10^9$/l).

Abnormal white cells of many forms may occur, but three important types form the large proportion of pathological leukocytes.

Myelocytes, primitive cells of the polymorphonuclear series, are normally present in the bone marrow but are present in the blood in large numbers in myelogenous leukaemia. A slightly more mature form, the metamyelocyte, may be seen up to a limit of 1 or 2 per cent in the blood of patients recently recovering from acute infections.

Myeloblasts are more primitive cells of the same series and may be seen in large numbers in acute myelogenous leukaemia and terminal chronic myelogenous leukaemia.

Lymphoblasts are the primitive form of the lymphocyte and appear in lymphatic leukaemia.

The presence of abnormal white cell forms is the warning sign of leukaemia, in some stages of which the total white count may be deceptively normal; therefore suspected blood disorders must be investigated by a differential white cell count as well as a total count. In these patients a platelet count is also essential (see below).

Investigation for Clotting Disorders
None of the tests previously described give any idea of the ability of the blood to form a clot. This is of obvious importance in dentistry and investigations must be carried out on all suspected "bleeders". It should always be remembered that haemostasis in any wound depends on capillary closure as well as on the coagulation properties of the blood. In cases in which the capillary mechanism is deficient, examination of the blood alone will give no hint of abnormality. For a simple screening procedure, estimations of the bleeding and clotting times are the most usual tests applied but, in fact, the information available as a result of these tests is minimal. For further investigation, more complex tests are needed.

Bleeding time.   In this test the lobe of the ear is punctured by a sharp lancet or the point of a scalpel. The precise nature of the puncture is not significant. The blood from the puncture is removed on filter paper every half minute until no further bleeding occurs. Normal values range from 2 to 3 minutes. These values - as are the values obtained for clotting times - are inaccurate and variable.

Clotting time.   Lee and White's method uses venous blood, 1 ml of which is placed in a tube 8 mm in internal diameter which is immersed in a water bath at $37^{o}C$. The tube is tilted from time to time and the clotting time is taken from the withdrawal of the blood to the time when the tube can be inverted without disturbing the clotted blood. The normal values range from 4 to 10 minutes at $37^{o}C$.

Wright's method consists of taking up blood obtained by puncture in a glass capillary tube some 1.5 mm in internal diameter. The tube is kept in a larger glass test-tube surrounded by a water bath at $37^{o}C$ and, at half-minute intervals, small pieces of the tube are broken off. When the blood has clotted, the broken ends of the tube are held together by a thread of clot. The time of this first occurring is noted. The clotting time obtained by this method has a normal variation of 6 to 10 minutes at $37^{o}C$.

Platelets (Thrombocytes).   Although the function of the platelets in the coagulation mechanism is not fully understood, it is
known that they play a vital part and that a reduction in their
number, as in a purpura, greatly increases the likelihood of
post-operative haemorrhage or of spontaneous bleeding.   Apart
from the significance of the platelet count in haemorrhagic
disorders it should be remembered that a reduction in platelet
numbers (thrombocytopenia) may occur in leukaemias and in some
other disturbances of haematopoesis such as aplastic anaemia.

    The platelets are technically difficult to count but they may
be directly counted in a chamber similar to that used for the
other blood constituents using a dilution of 1 in 200.   A common
diluting solution contains 3.8 per cent sodium citrate, 0.1 per
cent cresyl blue and 0.08 per cent formaldehyde, although several
other formulas of a similar type exist.   Mixing should be carried
out quickly to avoid clumping of the platelets and, after
settling, the count is made with a high power objective.

    The values for a normal adult range from 250,000 to 500,000
per mm^3 of blood.   (250-500 x 10^9l).

Capillary fragility test.   The tourniquet test gives some indication of either capillary incompetence or of great reduction in
platelet numbers.   An inflated cuff is applied to the upper arm,
maintained at 50 mm pressure of mercury for 15 minutes and then
released.   Normally a few small petechial haemorrhages will be
produced on the forearm (perhaps up to eight in number).   Many
petechiae, some of large size, however, strongly indicate a
disorder such as thrombocytopenic purpura.

    Should the screening tests show some disorder in the haemo-
static mechanism then steps must be taken to further determine
the nature of the defect.   On the whole, defects in the capillary
and platelet systems are shown up by the bleeding time estimation, a platelet count and a tourniquet test.   Examination for
further coagulation disorders includes tests to determine the
nature of the thromboplastin-prothrombin reaction in the individual patient.   Should defects be shown, then a whole series of
specific tests is available to show deficiencies in the coagulation mechanism.

Prothrombin
    Of these deficient factors that of factor II, prothrombin, is
probably the most common, and a determination of the amount of
prothrombin present in the blood is a common addition to the
specified screening tests.   The tests are devised to measure the
capacity of the plasma to clot in the presence of normal tissue
exudates.   In Quick's method excess thromboplastin (including a
platelet substitute) is added to the oxalated or citrated plasma
under test.   Excess of a calcium salt is then added in order to
neutralize the effect of the oxalate or citrate ions and to
provide calcium ions for the coagulation procedure.   The time
between the addition of the calcium salt solution and the formation of a firm clot is the prothrombin time (P.T.).   The normal

value is from 12 to 14 seconds and may be expressed in this way
or as a percentage value of the normal, taken as 12 seconds.

Partial Thromboplastin Time (P.T.T.). In this test a platelet
substitute (an incomplete thromboplastin) alone is added to the
recalcified plasma - no other thromboplastin constituents are
added and so the test is very sensitive to the presence, or
otherwise, of these factors. The clotting time is therefore
prolonged in a number of deficiency states including Factor VIII
deficiency (haemophillia) and Factor IX deficiency (Christmas
disease). The normal P.T.T. is taken as about 76 seconds, minor
variations depending on the precise reagents used. This test,
and prothrombin time estimations are now commonly carried out in
apparatus which automatically detects the onset of coagulation.

Serum Iron
    The great proportion of iron in the circulating blood is
combined as haemoglobin within the erythrocytes. A small
proportion, however, circulates in the serum, bound to a protein
transferin. This serum iron is the transport iron made available for haemoglobin synthesis from the body stores where it is
bound to another protein - ferritin. If the ferritin-bound body
stores become depleted there is a period of deficiency before
the haemoglobin levels begin to fall - this is sideropaenia or
latent iron deficiency. Oral symptoms may occur at this stage.
Estimations may be made of the serum iron itself and of the iron
binding components of the serum, (in iron deficiency the total
iron binding capacity or T.I.B.C. is often increased). From
these figures the percentage iron saturation of the serum may be
calculated. Normal values of serum iron are accepted as being
from 16 - 32 µmol/l, T.I.B.C. 64 - 106 µmol/l, and normal saturation as being over 16%. This last figure, now generally
accepted, is much lower than that normally adopted with older
methods of assessment than those now current.

Serum Vitamin B12
    Vitamin B12 is essential for the maintenance of effective
erythrocyte production - in its deficiency a megaloblastic
marrow results in the development of a macrocytic anaemia.   B12
is absorbed in the lower gut following conjugation with the
intrinsic factor produced in the gastric mucosa. Thus a
deficiency of B12 may result from either a dietary deficiency
(very rare), a lack of intrinsic factor (as in pernicious
anaemia or following gastrectomy) or in malabsorption states in
the lower gut.

    The initial test for B12 deficiency is an estimation of the
serum levels. The older test for this was a biological test,
depending on the enzymatic action of the vitamin in bacterial
growth processes. This has now been replaced by a radioimmune
assay process. In this method the serum, together with a known
quantity of radioactive labelled B12 is reacted with a previously prepared antigen. The proportion of radioactive mole-
cules in the final complex is measured and hence the proportion
of B12 added from the serum can be calculated. This, like many
other radioimmune assays may be carried out to a high degree of

accuracy. Normal serum values are of the order of 300 - 1,000
pg/ml (ng/l).

Folic Acid

Folic acid is also a factor necessary to prevent the onset of
megaloblastic anaemia. Apart from deficiencies due to pregnancy
and to the taking of anticonvulsant drugs such as epanutin
(phenytoin) the two common causes of folate deficiency are
dietary (often due to excessive alcohol intake) and malabsorption
due to pathological changes in the lower gut. Just as in the
case of B12 estimations, the older techniques were microbiolog-
ical, the newer ones are radioimmune assays. The normal values
are 3 - 200 ng/ml (µg/l). As in the case of B12 values, the
range of "normals" will vary from laboratory to laboratory,
depending on the precise methods used.

Sickle Cell Diseases

This is a genetically determined group of diseases in which
an abnormal haemoglobin (HbS) is present in the erythrocytes.
This form of haemoglobin occurs in many patients of negroid or
mediterranean ancestry and in some from the Middle and Far East.
When there is oxygen lack (as there may be, for example, in
anaesthesia) the erythrocytes take on a distorted 'sickle' shape.
There are two forms of the condition:-

   (a) sickle cell trait - inherited from one parent
        and implying deficient oxygen carrying capacity
        of the blood during oxygen lack (e.g. during
        anaesthesia). The patients are usually other-
        wise completely healthy.

   (b) sickle cell disease - inherited from both
        parents and in which there is permanent deficiency
        of the erythrocytes - this is highly unlikely to
        be first diagnosed as a dental problem.

The sickle cell trait is diagnosed simply by a slide test for
the presence of HbS. This test - the 'Sickledex Test' depends
on an erythrocyte clumping phenomenon when chemically deoxygen-
ated. This test should be performed on the blood of all 'at
risk' patients before general anaesthesia.

Erythrocyte Sedimentation Rate

In varying pathological processes the tendency of the erythrocytes to sediment from oxalated, citrated or heparinized blood
is accelerated. The mechanisms involved are not understood, but
it is thought that the properties of the plasma proteins may be
the deciding factors in this process. The method used is
usually that of Westergren in which 4.5 ml of venous blood are
mixed with 0.5 ml of 3.8 per cent sodium citrate solution. This
is transferred to a calibrated narrow bore glass tube and the
level of the sedimented red cells in 1 hour is read off directly.
The normal findings are from 0 to 15 mm in 1 hour in males, 0 to
20 mm in 1 hour in females. This rate may be much increased in
chronic inflammatory processes, in malignancy and during acute
infections.

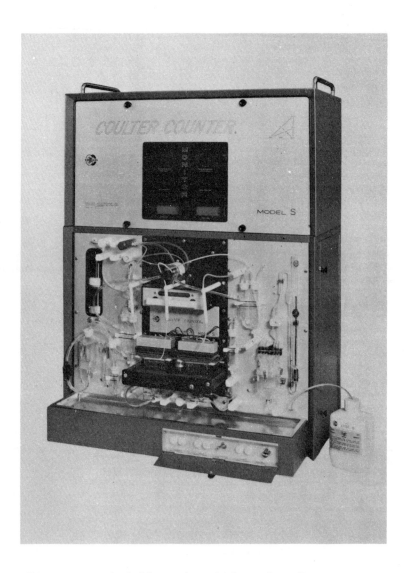

Fig. 2.1. A fully automated system for
carrying out full blood counts (the Coulter
Counter Model S). With apparatus of this kind
a complete report on cellular and platelet
content of the blood can be produced rapidly
from a single sample.

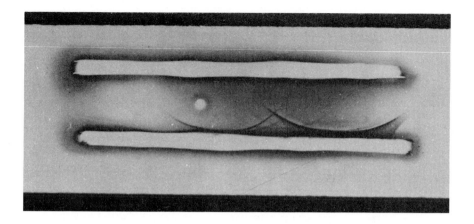

Fig. 2.2. Immuno-electrophoresis pattern produced during separation of plasma proteins. Each
arc represents a separate protein. The potential difference is applied along the long axis
of the plate whilst the serum diffuses from the
circular well.

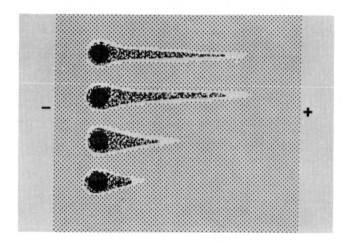

Fig. 2.3. Diagram of gel plate for quantitative
estimation of plasma proteins by immuno-
electrophoresis. The antigen is incorporated
into the gel itself and the length of the
'rockets' produced is related to the concentration of the protein in the serum placed in the
wells.

Bone Marrow Biopsy

In order to confirm or extend the information given by examination of the blood film, examination of the developing cells
of the marrow may be undertaken. The marrow is usually taken
from the sternum at a level between the second and third ribs.
Under local anaesthesia a wide bore needle is inserted into the
marrow cavity and a few drops of the marrow aspirated.

Films are prepared as in the case of blood, and stained in
the same way. Examination of these films is a procedure which
depends largely for its value on the experience of the investigator, differential counts being difficult to standardize. In
the proper hands, however, marrow biopsy can give vital information which may be obtained in no other manner. The distribution
of developing cell types may show distinctive arrangements in
leukaemias (even when aleukaemic, and hence difficult to diagnose
from blood films) and in pernicious and similar anaemias. Malignant cells from metastatic growths or multiple myeloma may be
found in the marrow, as may the typical "L.E." cells of disseminated lupus erythematosis. Variations in the formation of the
erythrocytes are also elucidated by marrow biopsy; for instance,
the macrocytic anaemias are most commonly finally diagnosed
following marrow examination.

The Plasma Proteins

Normal blood plasma contains 6 to 8 g of protein per 100 ml.
Of this albumins account for 3.5 to 5.6 g and the globulins 1.3
to 3.2 g, giving an albumin/globulin ratio of 1.5:1 to 2.5:1.
The total protein present may be determined chemically by a
colorimetric method which may easily be adapted to automatic
measurement. The total protein measured in this way has a wide
variety of components each with differing functions. Many of
these vary in concentration and composition during disease. The
earlier division of plasma proteins into alpha, beta and gamma
globulins and albumin, although chemically accurate is a somewhat
gross division with respect to pathological and physiological
changes and it is only with the advance of techniques able to
separate the minor constituents from these broad divisions that
useful diagnostic tests have become available. Quantitization
of the serum proteins is now routinely carried out by immuno-
chemical techniques, some of which have considerable value in
the diagnosis of oral disease. This is particularly true in the
case of the immunoglobulins.

With a greater understanding of the function of the lymphocytes in the two branches of the immune response (cell mediated
and humoral) together with the existence of co-ordinating
systems (such as transfer factor) methods have also been developed for an assessment of lymphocyte activity in differing
pathological conditions.

Immunological Investigations

A large and increasing number of techniques are available for
the study of patients with suspected immune defects. In the

present context it is possible only to briefly mention a few of
those most likely to be of use in the investigation of patients
seen in the oral medicine clinic.

(1) Gell diffusion techniques for the separation of
plasma proteins. These depend on the differing rates of diffusion of substances of different molecular weights through gell
media. If, for example, a mixture of plasma proteins is placed
in a well cut into an agar gell plate, each will diffuse out at
a different rate and by "developing" the resulting rings in the
gell by precipitation with a suitable antigen it is possible to
assay the various constituents of the mixture. This may be the
basis of either a qualitative or a quantitative test, depending
on the precise method used. An elaboration of this method is
that of immunoelectrophoresis, a process often used for the
separation of the components of human serum. The principle is
as follows: The serum is placed in a well in an agar gell plate
through which diffusion occurs. In this case the process is not
of simple diffusion since an electric potential difference is
induced across the gell. The rates of diffusion of the various
proteins are therefore determined not only by such factors as
molecular weight but also by their electrochemical properties.
Following this electrophoretic separation a solution containing
suitable antigens is allowed to diffuse through the gell in a
direction at right angles to the axis along which the potential
difference has been applied. An antibody - antigen reaction
takes place and characteristic precipitation arcs are formed in
the gell (Fig. 2.2). There are many possible refinements and
modifications of the technique - a wide range of gell plates is
available and the development of the characteristic patterns may
be shown by the use of various antigens, chemical reactants and
stains which may be included in the gell itself, thus simplifying
the procedure (Fig. 2.3). Radio-immuno assay may also be used
for the differentiation of immunoglobulins and is in fact a
highly sensitive method. However, as yet the diffusion techniques are more commonly available.

(2) A wide range of methods is available for the detection and estimation of specific antibodies - particularly those
produced in response to infection. These, although technically
quite complex, are much more routinely performed than the other
investigations outlined here, and are available in a considerable
number of laboratories. The various serological tests for
syphilis come into this category, as do the estimations of antiviral antibodies in serum. Often, as in the cases mentioned,
these serological tests may be the only means available for
accurate identification of the infective agent. They are further
discussed in Chapter 3.

(3) The identification of T and B lymphocytes. This is
dependent largely on their immunological characteristics,
although, as previously mentioned there are ultrastructural
differences between lymphocytes of the two types. An example of
the type of method used to differentiate the groups is shown in
Fig. 2.4 in which erythrocytes are seen surrounding a T lymphocyte previously sensitised to erythrocyte surface antigen. For

the separation of the T and B lymphocytes on a larger scale
diffusion techniques have been evolved in which the immunological
characteristics of the cells are employed to effect the separation. However, it cannot be said at the present time that tests
designed to separate and enumerate T and B lymphocytes are part
of normal laboratory investigations - they are at present largely
a research weapon.

    (4) The lymphocyte transformation test. This demon-
strates the transformation of sensitised T lymphocytes into the
lymphoblast form when again stimulated by the sensitising antigen. Lymphoblastic transformation and proliferation can be
measured by carrying out the transformation in a medium containing
radioactively labelled thymidine (an aminoacid which is incorporated into nuclei during mitosis). In this way the nuclei of
the transformed cells themselves become radioactively labelled
and can be detected by the use of a photographic emulsion deposited over a microscopic preparation of the cells (Fig. 2.5).

    (5) The lymphokynes released during lymphocytic trans-
formation can be detected by suitable methods. For example, the
migration inhibition factor may be assessed by measuring the
rate of migration of macrophages from a capillary tube placed in
a medium containing the secreted factor. Similar biochemical
assay methods are available for other lymphokynes.

    (6) Immunofluorescence. This is perhaps the most elegant
method of demonstrating antibody formation and fixation onto
tissue and is of great value in the study of autoimmune mechanisms. The principle of this technique depends on the fact that
antibodies combined with fluoroscein retain both their immunological activity and the ability of the fluoroscein to fluoresce
under ultra violet light. Because of this antibodies can be
located at their exact site of combination with their antigenic
antagonists by microscopic observation under ultra violet illumination. There are two basic methods available. The first of
these is the direct method in which specific antibody must be
prepared, conjugated with fluoroscein and then reacted on a
microscope slide against a section of the tissue involved.
Examples of this are shown in Figs. 2.6, 2.7 in which the presence of antibody - antigen reaction sites is demonstrated in
different epithelial structures in pemphigus and pemphigoid.
The second method (the indirect method) can perhaps be best
illustrated by a specific example - the investigation of patients
with Sjögren's syndrome for antibodies directed against salivary
gland tissue. In this case normal salivary gland tissue, taken
from a subject without disease, is reacted with the serum from
the patient under investigation. The antibody in the serum is
then able to react with the antigens of the salivary gland tissue
and becomes fixed to it. This antibody (an IgG) is then marked
by adding antihuman IgG (produced in animals) labelled with
fluoroscein. Again, this is carried out on a microscope slide
and the site of the antibody - antigen reaction is shown by
examination under ultra violet light.

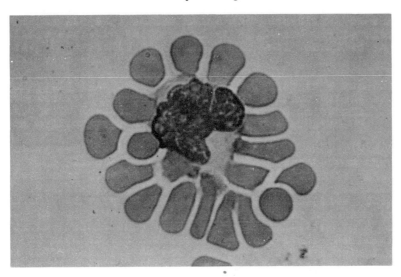

Fig. 2.4. A T-lymphocyte surrounded by erythrocytes. The lymphocyte had previously been
sensitized to erythrocyte surface antigen.

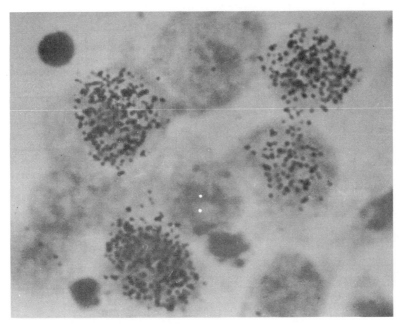

Fig. 2.5. Lymphoblast transformation and
proliferation. The nuclei of the activated
cells are labelled with radioactive Thymidine.

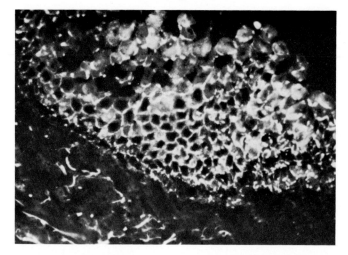

Fig. 2.6. Immunofluorescent labelling of antibodies present in pemphigus. In this case the
specific antibodies are present around and
between the cells of the prickle cell layer of
the epithelium.

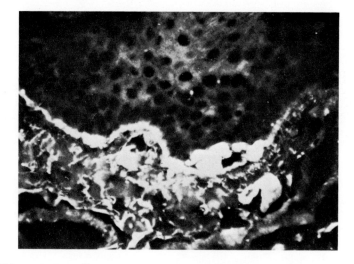

Fig. 2.7. Immunofluorescent labelling of antibodies in pemphigoid. In this condition the
antibodies are seen at and around the basal
complex.

It is evident that none of these methods of immunological
investigation are simple and most of them are available only in
highly specialised laboratories at the present time. However, in
certain cases, the kind of investigations described may be of
great importance in assessing pathological processes of the oral
mucosa.

Specific Diagnostic Tests

In a number of disease processes specific proteins may be
detected in the serum. A number of diagnostic tests have been
devised based on the detection of such specific proteins. Some
of these are available as slide tests, the reaction taking place
on the surface of a ready prepared glass slide using minimal
quantities of serum and of reagents.

R.A. factor (rheumatoid arthritis)
In rheumatoid arthritis a group of proteins specific to the
disease appears in the serum. These are known as rheumatoid
arthritis factor or rheumatoid factor and are present in a large
proportion of patients with the disease from an early stage. It
is thought that the R.A. factor proteins are antibodies against
abnormal gamma globulins.

The test commonly used is a latex agglutination test depending
on a reaction between the serum and an immunoglobulin coated onto
extremely finely dispersed polystyrene latex particles. The
serum under test is mixed with the reagent and separate positive
and negative controls are also tested at the same time. A positive result is indicated by clumping and agglutination of the
latex particles.

C-reactive protein (C.R.P.)
C-reactive protein is of unknown function but appears in the
sera of patients undergoing acute inflammatory reactions and in
some other conditions such as rheumatoid arthritis. The tests
devised for the demonstration of C-reactive protein exactly
parallel those used for R.A. factor. A similar latex suspension
is used, the particles in this case being coated with an antihuman C-reactive protein of animal origin. A positive result is
indicated by agglutination (Fig. 2.8).

Lupus Erythematosus Factor (L.E.F.)
In lupus erythematosus a specific serum factor is present in a
large proportion of cases. It represents one of a number of antibodies found in the serum of these patients. Again, a slide test
is available based on agglutination but in this case sensitised
erythrocytes are more often used as indicators of the reaction.
This test is often used as a screening procedure before carrying
out the more complex search for the characteristic leucocytes
found in the condition (the L.E. cells). These L.E. cells
consist of polymorphs which have phagocytosed cells which have
themselves been damaged by anti-nuclear antibodies. The resulting L.E. cells contain amorphous basophilic bodies which are
effectively specific for lupus erythematosus.

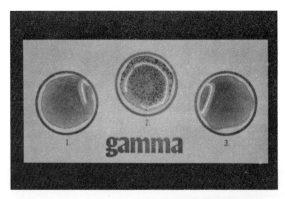

Fig. 2.8.   Slide test for C-reactive
protein.   The agglutination of the
positive control serum on plate 2 is
evident, Plate 1 contains the serum
under test and plate 3 the negative
control serum.   This represents a
negative result.

Anti-nuclear factor
      Anti-nuclear factor (ANF) is one of a number of antibodies
which may be found in a wide range of diseases - particularly
those with an autoimmune basis.   These autoantibodies include
those to D.N.A., gastric epithelial cells, salivary duct cells
and to other specific tissues.   Often a number of these autoantibodies are present in a single disease, the highest concentration being of that associated with the most severely affected
organ.   Thus it is usual to carry out a series of tests rather
than a single specific one.   Immunofluorescent methods are used
and have become much more specific with the gradual introduction
of satisfactory reagents capable of standardisation.

      Anti-nuclear factor may be present (together with other auto-
antibodies) in a variable proportion of patients with the following conditions which might be related to oral disease:-
systemic lupus erythematosus, rheumatoid arthritis, chronic
discoid lupus, Sjögren's syndrome, ulcerative colitis.   It is
not found in rheumatic fever.   Tissue specific autoantibodies may
be found in Addison's disease, pernicious anaemia, ulcerative
colitis and Sjögren's syndrome amongst others.

      The precise function of the autoantibodies is not known.

Chemical Examination of the Blood
    Blood chemistry determinations are taken to include the anal-
ysis of the non-protein and inorganic constituents of the blood.
Those normally called for in oral diagnostic procedures are of
calcium, phosphorus and alkaline phosphatase.

    Estimations of this kind, until relatively recently carried
out by laborious chemical and biochemical techniques, are now
universally carried out in automatic equipment of a wide range
of design. Colorimetric, fluorescent and immunological methods
represent some of the techniques used in this field and the
equipment is often of a high degree of sophistication. As in the
case of the automated blood counting equipment mentioned above,
it is common to find equipment designed to carry out a whole
range of tests on a single specimen of blood, the results being
automatically printed out in a very short time. This represents
a tremendous technical advance over the old time-consuming
methods.

    The estimations of the serum concentrations of calcium, phos-
phorus (as inorganic phosphate) and alkaline phosphatase are
carried out by colorimetric methods, most commonly in one of the
multi-functional machines described above. The normal values
for serum calcium remains relatively constant in respect of age
and sex from between 8.5 to 11.5 mg per 100 ml serum (S.I. units
2.3 - 2.7 m.mol/l). The determination of phosphorus (as inorganic phosphate) is also carried out colorimetrically and by a
parallel process to that for calcium. Normal values range from
2.5 to 5 mg per 100 ml in adults (0.8 - 1.6 m.mol/l) and from
4 to 7 milligrammes per 100 ml in children (1.3 to 2.3 m.mol/l).

    The S.I. units adopted for alkaline phosphatase (international
units - I.U.) are unfortunately arbitrary units with no greater
fundamental basis than those of the previously used King Armstrong or Bodansky units. The conversion from international
units to King Armstrong units is non linear. It should be
realised that enzyme assay methods are highly dependent on the
precise technique employed and thus the various units may not be
directly comparable by means of a simple conversion factor. For
the interpretation of figures such as these the laboratory should
be contacted if any doubt exists and the normal values associated
with the precise method used should be ascertained. In most laboratories adult values of up to 375 I.U. may be expected. They
are higher in children and at adolescence.

Plasma Glucose
    The assessment of plasma glucose levels plays an occasional
part in the screening of patients who may have oral symptoms
related to diabetes mellitus or incipient diabetes. The tests
used depend on the reducing properties of the blood sugar, the
determinations being almost universally automated. Venous blood
is usually used and is collected into a tube containing sodium
fluoride as a preservative. The normal values quoted for plasma
glucose (60-120 mg/100 ml, 3.5 - 7 m mol/l) must be treated with
caution. There is considerable variation according to the precise time of day and, according to the amount of dietary

carbohydrate ingested by the patient. The diagnosis of diabetes
is made following a provocative test in which the response of the
homeostatic mechanisms to a single large dose of glucose is
measured. A fasting glucose estimation is followed by the administration orally of 50 grams of glucose and the subsequent rise
in the blood glucose level is measured every half hour for the
subsequent two hours. At the same time urinary glucose output is
qualitatively measured. In this way the effectiveness of the
insulin response is shown by the behaviour of the blood glucose
levels and an indication of the renal threshold is given according to a point at which urinary overspill of glucose takes place.
It should be emphasised that carefully controlled conditions are
necessary to provide reproducible results in the glucose tolerance test.

    It should be added that a simple and rapid rough test has
been devised using an indicator paper on which a single drop of
blood is used. The colour developed is compared with a standard
chart and the glucose values may be estimated.

Plasma Cortisol
    The determination of plasma cortisol (the naturally occurring
cortico-steroid with similar properties to hydrocortizone) is
carried out by a specific fluoresence test. Normal values are
given as between 7 and 25 µg/100 ml (140 - 700 n mol/l) but,
rather as in the case of plasma glucose, these figures are liable
to considerable variation under normal circumstances. In order
to assess adrenal response it is necessary to stimulate the
natural production of cortisol and to follow the resultant blood
levels over a period of some hours. The stimulation is normally
carried out by the use of a small dose of Synacthen (a synthetic
analogue of A.C.T.H.). In a normal response the base line level
of cortisol is at least doubled in approximately one hour. If
the adrenal function is inhibited either by a disease process or
by long continued steroid therapy, this response is deficient.
Just as in the glucose tolerance test the precise conditions of
the Synacthen stimulation test are of vital importance in attain-
ing reproducible results.

                                Urine

    The composition of urine is complex. It consists of an
aqueous solution of many metabolic by-products which vary considerably in composition and concentration in disease. Its daily
volume is normally of the order of 1500 ml in adults.

    Indicator papers have been produced which, simply dipped into
the urine sample, give colour reactions not only for pH, but also
for the presence of sugars, blood and proteins. These colour
changes are all roughly quantitative. These indicators are now
almost universally used for routine checking procedures, being
simple, reasonably accurate and capable of being used by non-
technical staff or even by the patient himself if need be.

    The routine hospital examination carried out as a screening

test for pathological changes in the urine is often referred to
as a M.S.S.U. test (midstream specimen of urine). In this case
the urine is collected so as to avoid the beginning and the end
of micturition. It is examined and reported on for colour, pH,
specific gravity, the presence of sugars and other reducing
substances, proteins and any crystalline or other solid substances, cells, casts, etc. The urine is also cultured and a
report on any bacteria present is given.

Traces of sugars may be present in urine in health, especially
after the ingestion of large quantities of carbohydrates. The
presence of any appreciable quantity of sugars is, however, of
pathological significance and thus a qualitative test only is
necessary to indicate some disorder. The report is given as
either trace, +, ++, or +++.

A similar convention is used to report on protein and on blood
in the urine.

Vitamins

Although a number of complex deficiencies (most often caused
by malabsorbtion in some form) may be reflected in oral changes
vitamin C deficiency is almost the only simple avitaminosis
encountered in dental surgery. Perhaps the best diagnostic test
for the deficiency is the extremely rapid reversal of clinical
symptoms on giving large doses of ascorbic acid to the patient.
If, however, a quantitative test is required, this may be carried
out by administering ascorbic acid intravenously and by measuring
the urinary output subsequently (normal adult excretion is about
25 mg/day). The technique of estimation is a complex but accurate one, utilizing a reaction in which a dye, 2-6-dichlorophenol-
indo-phenol, is quantitatively decolorized by reaction with
ascorbic acid. If the patient has a deficient intake of ascorbic
acid he will not rapidly excrete the given dose as do those
individuals normally nourished.

A similar technique can be used to measure the blood plasma
concentration of ascorbic acid. This is of the order of 8-14 mg
per 100 ml plasma in health.

A more accurate measure of the blood levels of ascorbic acid
is given by an estimation of the leukocyte acid level. A reduction in this figure (from the normal of over 20 $mg/10^8$ leukocytes) is a better indication of a deficiency than is a reduction in the somewhat labile plasma concentration. As in other
biochemical determinations it is essential to know the usual
normal values for the laboratory concerned.

Methods have been developed for the estimation of blood or
urinary levels of thiamine (B1), riboflavine (B2), nicotinic
acid and pyridoxine (B6). A number of colorimetric and chromat-
ographic methods may be used, but these are available only in
specialised laboratories and are very rarely called for in the
diagnosis of oral disease.

TABLE IV

HAEMATOLOGICAL VALUES

	Old unit	S.I. unit	Conversion Factors S.I. to old	S.I. Normal Values
Erythrocytes (RBC)	$/mm^3$	/1	$\times 10^{-6}$	$4.5-6.5 \times 10^{12}$ /1
Leukocytes (WBC)	"	"	"	$4-11 \times 10^9$/1
Platelets	"	"	"	$150-400 \times 10^9$/1
Haemoglobin	g/100ml	g/dl	$\times 1$	14.4g/dl
Iron (Serum)	μg/100ml	μmol/1	$\times 5.58$	13-32
Iron Binding Capacity	"	"	$\times 5.58$	64-106
Folate	ng/ml	μg/1	$\times 1$	3-20
B_{12}	pg/ml	ng/1	$\times 1$	300-1,000
Glucose	mg/100ml	nmol/1	$\times 18$	3.5-7.5 nmol/1
Calcium	mg/100ml	nmol/1	$\times 4.0$	2.2-2.7
Alkaline Phosphatase	King Armstrong	I.U./1		Variable, (see below)
Phosphate	mg/100ml	nmol/1	$\times 3.1$	0.8-1.4
Cortisol	μg/100ml	nmol/1	$\times .036$	140-500 (Fasting 9.00 a.m.)

The 'normal' values may vary according to the technique used and should always be determined.

The values for Alkaline Phosphatase are particularly dependant on the technique. The conversion is non linear.

Chapter III

Biopsy and Bacteriology

Biopsy

Many lesions may be diagnosed only after examination of an appropriate biopsy specimen of the affected tissue. This is so, not only in cases of suspected neoplasia, but, for example, in the differential diagnosis of white patches which may occur in the oral mucosa and of the bullous, ulcerative and desquamative lesions in the mouth. Many bone conditions are similarly only capable of final diagnosis by examination of a biopsy sample. It is generally agreed that, in the case of suspected or possible malignancy of the oral mucosa, biopsy is mandatory and with simple precautions is unlikely to cause dissemination of tumour cells. There are several methods of obtaining biopsies and these will be dealt with under the following headings: smear, excisional, incisional, aspiration and bone.

Smear Biopsy

The examination of vaginal smears is well recognized as of great help in the diagnosis of early uterine and cervical carcinoma. Similarly much progress has been made in the recognition of malignant cells, floating free in various body fluids, which originate from otherwise undetectable neoplasms.

This success in the recognition of desquamated tumour cells does not extend to malignant lesions of the oral epithelium. Smears taken directly from the surface of proved malignancies may well show only keratinized squames in the light microscope and give no indication of the nature of the lesion. Thus it should be categorically stated that exfoliative cytology has no place in the routine diagnosis of suspected oral malignancy. It is always necessary to carry out biopsy of the excisional or incisional type and the accessibility of the oral mucosa makes this a relatively simple procedure. It is interesting to note that recent work has shown that scanning electron microscopy of cells exfoliated from oral malignancies may demonstrate characteristic morphological changes which may eventually be of use in diagnosis. However, this is as yet a completely undeveloped technique.

A study of epithelial smears may be of great value in the differential diagnosis of the bullous and other similar lesions of the oral mucosa. The technique adopted is to scrape gently the surface of the affected area with a fairly broad square-ended instrument such as a spatula. (No preliminary cleansing of the area should be carried out.) The smear is transferred directly to a previously cleaned slide, spread into a thin film by the spatula and immediately fixed by dropping into 50 per cent ether-

ethyl alcohol. If more than one area is to be studied, the spatula must either be carefully cleaned or replaced before the next
smear is taken. If an intact bulla is available then the fluid
contents should be aspirated and spread on the slide which is
fixed in the same way. After fixing for a minimum of 10 minutes,
the slides may be stained. For purposes of oral diagnosis,
haematoxylin and eosin is probably best, the complex stain specified by Papanicolaou for the study of cervical smears being
somewhat less successful for oral conditions. A valuable alternative method of fixation is by the use of one of the commercially
available spray products packed in pressurized containers and
originally intended for use in cervical cytology. These are much
more convenient than the highly inflammable ether-alcohol mixture.

Smear cytology may also be of value in the diagnosis of oral
infections and is discussed below.

After mounting the slides, the whole of the smear should be
carefully surveyed in an orderly manner, scanning one field
width at a time until the whole smear has been seen under first
low and then high power. This is necessary as the abnormal cells
upon which the diagnosis depends may be few in number and may be
accompanied by many cells of normal appearance. (Many oral
smears show great numbers of polymorphs present, together with
the epithelial cells.) Figure 3.1 shows an oral smear from a
case of pemphigus - a condition in which the fragile nature of
the bullae produced makes incisional or excisional biopsy very
difficult. When taking samples from ruptured bullae an attempt
should be made to obtain epithelial cells from the edge of the
area - the centre of the eroded area is likely to yield a great
majority of inflammatory cells.

Only positive results can be accepted in oral exfoliative
cytology - essentially normal findings should be confirmed by
further methods.

Excisional Biopsy
    If the lesion in question is small, it may be best to remove
it entirely by local excision, including a small area of normal
tissue. The specimen may then be sectioned and its histology
reviewed to determine whether further treatment will be needed.
The biopsy is far better taken with the knife than with the
cutting diathermy which may cause considerable distortion of the
tissues. If diathermy is felt necessary, as in a suspected
malignancy, then the operation bed can be coagulated after the
excision.

After its removal, the biopsy specimen should be placed with
the minimum of delay into a fixative, 10 per cent formol saline
being the most universally used. Full clinical details should
always be given to the pathologist who is to study the specimen.

Excision biopsy is particularly useful for the diagnosis of
single small ulcers and small localized soft tissue swellings.
In these cases it is virtually equivalent to combining primary
treatment with biopsy.

A special case occurs in the use of cryosurgery for the treatment of potentially malignant, highly vascular or similar lesions. The problem is that the whole of the tissue treated is lost by sloughing and is thus not available for histological study. In these circumstances a biopsy specimen may be removed from the area when frozen with little fear of haemorrhage or other troublesome complication. If it is thought essential the whole of the frozen lesion can be removed in this way, combining some of the advantages of cryosurgery with those of biopsy excision.

Incisional Biopsy
This is the removal of a section of a lesion for histological study without any attempt being made to remove the whole of the lesion. In taking such a biopsy of the oral soft tissues, an attempt should be made to include within one specimen, if possible, a clinically typical area of the lesion and also the edge of the lesion. If the choice must be made between the two possibilities, the clinically typical area should be chosen; a large area of normal tissue beyond the lesion is quite unnecessary. The specimen should be big enough to give the pathologist a reasonable chance to make a diagnosis, as too small a biopsy is difficult to handle and to orient for sectioning.

The technique for biopsy of a lesion of the oral epithelium, is to make a wedge-shaped cut into the chosen area, to complete the triangle by a third cut and to then take off the epithelial layer, together with a thickness of corium, by sliding the knife below and parallel with the surface. Even if it is the epithelium which is of particular interest, it is essential that a sufficient layer of corium should be included in order that the subepithelial reactions may be seen. If the biopsy is of a lump, then the wedge section must be taken into the swelling, making sure that any capsular tissue is cut through, and a representative area of the lesion proper is obtained.

Anaesthesia for the biopsy should be obtained by the injection of local anaesthetic as far from the biopsy site as consistent with obtaining a satisfactory result. It is clearly unwise to inject directly into an area of doubtful malignancy, and quite apart from any question of dissemination of neoplastic cells, there is a danger of distortion of the histological picture if the area is locally infiltrated by anaesthetic. The biopsy site may be closed by one or two silk sutures.

If the specimen is a thin one, as is often the case with biopsies of the oral mucosa, it is often most convenient to lay it flat on a piece of card or a swab before dropping into the fixative. The tissue practically always adheres to this backing and curling and distortion of the specimen is prevented.

Frozen sections are rarely required in oral surgical practice - very often the specimens obtained by biopsy are in need of careful and detailed study, this being very difficult with frozen tissue. On rare occasions, however, when an urgent decision is essential on some major point (for example, whether a lesion is

malignant or not) then a rapid result is obtained by cutting
sections on a freezing microtome. Stained sections can be reported on in a very short time - of the order of a few minutes.
The most usual form of apparatus depends on the cooling effect of
a jet of carbon dioxide. On the whole, however, the sections are
poor, the procedure is disliked by pathologists and it is advisable to ask for frozen sections only when essential.

Aspiration Biopsy

Aspiration biopsy, that is the removal of fluid or semi-fluid
material from the tissues by an aspirating syringe, has some
uses in oral diagnosis. It is of particular value in disting-
uishing a fluid filled cystic cavity from a solid lesion, or
from an air filled one (such as the antrum). The technique is
simple, the main difficulty which may arise being due to the use
of too fine a needle; this preferably should not be less than 14
gauge. In most sites a few drops of local anaesthetic only are
needed to make the process quite painless. The most usual indication for aspiration biopsy at the present time is in the differentiation of the various types of odontogenic cyst and, in
particular, the identification of the keratocyst by analysis of
the cyst fluid constituents. This technique will be further
discussed in the appropriate section of chapter VII.

A specially important use of aspiration biopsy occurs in the
identification of blood filled lesions - in particular, of central haemangiomas. These lesions (also further discussed in
chapter VII) are extremely dangerous if approached surgically
without having been identified, and any doubtful lesion which
might come into this group should be aspirated. However, it
should be realised that even this measure is not without danger,
since persistent bleeding may occur from the aspiration site -
in one reported case this was fatal.

Bone Biopsy

In the diagnosis of lesions of bone, a biopsy is often helpful. This may be obtained, after raising a soft tissue flap,
with a chisel, but the process can be facilitated by the use of
a specially designed bone biopsy drill. This drill, in the form
of a hollow cylinder is fitted into a straight dental handpiece
and, after raising a small muco-periosteal flap, can be entered
to its full depth into the bone. A slight lateral movement is
sufficient to separate the cut cylinder of bone at its base when
it may be removed within the drill. The bone is then pushed out
from the drill into the fixative and the flap closed by silk
sutures.

Before sections of bone may be stained and examined, they
must be decalcified, a process which takes a considerable time -
usually at least a week even in a fast decalcifying agent such
as aqueous nitric acid. In general the greater the rate of
decalcification, the greater the risk of distortion of the tissues in the process and, unless the need is urgent, some little
time should be allowed for the processing of a bone specimen.

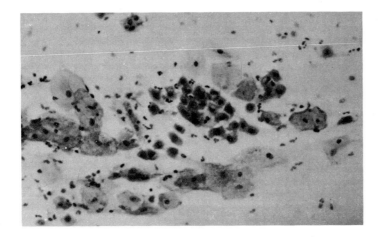

Fig. 3.1.   Smear from a bulla in a case of
pemphigus.   The rounded hyperchromic acantholytic cells are typical of the condition and are
accompanied in this field by relatively normal
epithelial cells and many inflammatory cells.

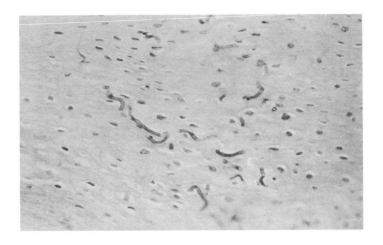

Fig. 3.2.   Candida albicans penetrating the
epithelium in a case of candidal leukoplakia
(P.A.S. stain).

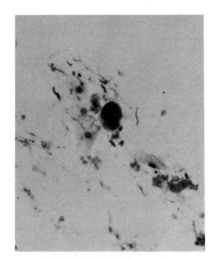 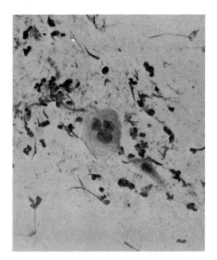

Fig. 3.3. A cell containing inclusion bodies
(left) and a multinucleated epithelial cell
(right) from a smear in acute herpetic stomatitis.

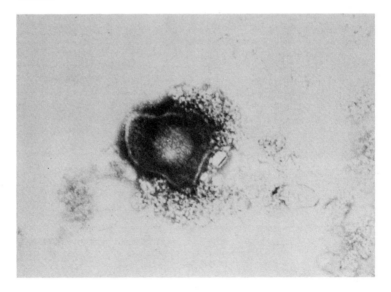

Fig. 3.4. Electron micrograph of a viral particle from a case of herpes simplex (x 140k).

Bacteriological Investigation

If a bacterial infection is present or suspected, then swabs may be taken from the area and the organism involved isolated and tested for antibiotic sensitivity. In most oral diagnostic procedures, the swab is taken directly from the affected area with considerable care being taken to avoid contamination from any source. It is almost impossible to eliminate normal oral organisms by the use of surface antiseptics round about the swabbed area and their use is contra-indicated. After taking the infected matter up on the swab, it should be carefully placed in its sterile glass tube, together with its cotton-wool cap, great care being taken not to touch the tube rim with the swab. If the conditions are such that an aspirated specimen of pus may be safely obtained, then there is much more certainty of an uncontaminated sample. However, not many infected lesions can be treated in this way.

On arrival at the laboratory the swab should be smeared directly on to a sterile microscope slide, then on to two blood agar plates, finally being dropped into a broth medium. The smeared slide is stained by Gram's stain and examined at once. On this smear for example may be seen the overwhelming growth of fusiform and spirochaetal organisms present in a Vincent's infection. These organisms will not be shown up in the subsequent cultures, as special techniques are required for their growth.

The two inoculated blood plates are incubated for 24 hours, one aerobically, the other anaerobically. The colonies appearing are identified and the organisms transferred to other plates on the surface of which are placed paper test discs impregnated with small standard quantities of various antibodies. A further 24 hours' incubation gives growth except in the vicinity of antibiotics to which the organisms are sensitive.

The inoculated broth may be used to show up organisms difficult to culture directly on plates or which were scanty on the original swab.

The completed report on the swab will consist of three parts; the results of direct smear examination, the organisms cultured and identified, and their antibiotic sensitivities. If further information is required or special culture techniques are felt to be necessary, as for the tubercle bacillus, then these must be specifically asked for.

Syphilis
Oral Syphilis is not a common condition but it is evidently of great importance that it should be recognised. A number of tests are available for laboratory diagnosis.

> 1. Dark ground examination of fluid from a primary
> or secondary lesion may demonstrate the presence of
> treponema pallidum. This may be the only available
> diagnostic method for early confirmation of a primary

lesion before antibody development has
occurred.

2.   Serological tests still form the basis of
the laboratory diagnosis of syphilis.   In the
first of these tests, developed by Wassermann,
the antibodies in the suspected blood or cerebro-
spinal fluid were brought into reaction with the
antigens in aqueous suspensions of syphilitic
tissues.   It was soon found, however, that the
reaction was, in fact, non-specific and that
alcoholic extracts of normal tissues could replace
the aqueous syphilitic suspension.   From this
observation a number of techniques have been
evolved, known as "complement fixation tests".
Complement is a substance present in normal
blood which takes part in a complementary
manner in the antigen-antibody reaction, reacting
itself with the antigen but only in the presence
of antibody.

   The Kahn test for syphilis, on the other hand,
is an example of a flocculation test in which the
antigen is added to the patient's serum and, if
antibodies are present, a precipitate is formed
by the reaction of the two.   The antigen is again
non-specific, being in the standard Kahn reaction
an alcoholic extract of beef heart.

   Since the technical details of the reactions
are complicated and lengthy the tests must be
carried out under fully standardized conditions.
For this reason, regional centres of investigation
are widely accepted as the best and most trustworthy
laboratories for the carrying out of these tests.
Material for the test consists of at least 10 ml
of venous blood delivered into a clear, dry,
sterile bottle.   It is general practice to carry
out both a complement fixation and a flocculation
test on each sample.   Results in each case are
reported as +++, ++, +, + or - depending on the
intensity of the reaction.   Negative results in
both complement fixation and flocculation tests,
repeated in each case after an interval of time,
may be considered a true negative.   Doubtful or
weak positive results must be repeated.

   In very early syphilis a negative reaction
to both tests is common.   Within a month of
primary infection, however, virtually all patients
show a positive reaction and this is maintained
into the secondary stage.   In untreated patients
with tertiary syphilis there may be occasional
false negative results.   False positives may be
given during febrile infections, particularly

infective mononucleosis (glandular fever),
but these are usually transient.

A number of variations of the original
tests have been devised, perhaps the most
widely used being the V.D.R.L. (Venereal
Disease Research Laboratory) test, which is
a flocculation test carried out on a slide.
This is considered to be reliable and
inexpensive. Most laboratories, however,
continue to perform at least two different
tests on each specimen.

3. Treponemal tests are increasingly used
in the diagnosis of more difficult cases.
In the treponema pallidum immobilisation
test (T.P.I.) live treponemal organisms are
exposed to the patient's serum. If antibodies
are present immobilisation of the motile
organisms occurs and is observed by dark field
microscopy.

A modified treponemal test which is being
increasingly used is based on immunofluorescence.
A slide with smeared known organisms is exposed
to the patient's serum. If antibodies are
present they become attached to the treponema
and may be shown up by treatment with a
fluorescein - antihuman globulin conjugate
which fluoresces brightly in the ultra violet
light microscope. This is the F.T.A. (fluorescent
treponemal antibody) or F.T.A. - A.B.S. test.

Tuberculosis
Oral tuberculosis is even less common than oral syphilis but
it is particularly important that it should be recognised.
Almost invariably the initial diagnosis is suggested by a tuber-
culoid histology following biopsy of a patch or ulcer of unknown
origin. Such a histology is, however, relatively non specific
and a firm diagnosis of tuberculosis depends on a demonstration
of acid fast organisms using the Ziehl-Neelsen staining technique.
In spite of repeated statements to the contrary it is not by any
means certain that these can be shown up in the affected tissue,
even with the most careful study. Similarly, superficial swabs
taken from an oral lesion may fail to yield organisms for culture. It is necessary to take further unfixed biopsy tissue from
the lesion which may be used, following mechanical disintegration,
as an innoculum for animal and in vitro studies. Animal innocu-
lation methods of this kind depend on the high susceptibility of
the rabbit or guinea-pig to human strains of the tubercle organisms.

Actinomycosis
Any chronic pyogenic process related to the oral cavity should
come under suspicion as possibly actinomycosis. If this is suspected a direct smear of the pus, examined by the naked eye, may

show up the classical "sulphur granules" consisting of clumps of
the organisms and low power magnification may indicate the masses
of radiating mycelia.   Confirmation may be made by culturing
anaerobically.   Immunofluorescent tests are available if required,
which enable the various serotypes to be differentiated.

Caries Susceptibility Tests

Several bacterial tests have been devised to measure the susceptibility of the individual to caries. Most of these depend on
the estimation of either the number or the activity of the acid
producing organisms present in the saliva. In the lactobacillus
test the saliva is collected by chewing paraffin wax immediately
after getting up in the morning. The saliva is then diluted and
the organisms inoculated on to a selective medium of tomato agar
at pH 5 and incubated for 96 hours. Counts of over 10,000 have a
moderate to marked caries activity, between 1,000 and 10,000
slight to moderate activity and below 1,000 very slight or none.

The Snyder test, the second of the commonly used tests for
caries susceptibility, consists of the inoculation of saliva into
a 2 per cent dextrose broth. The acid produced by the activity
of the organisms of the saliva is indicated by bromcresol green,
the time taken for the change being recorded. The more rapidly
the colour change occurs, the more actively caries-susceptible is
the subject.

These tests only provide a general picture of the susceptibility to caries and are mainly used for dental health educational
purposes.

Blood Cultures

The culture of organisms present in the blood is of great
importance in the diagnosis of many diffuse and widespread infections, although not commonly found necessary in oral diagnosis.
Blood cultures have, however, been widely carried out in the
study of the transient bacteriaemias provoked by dental treatment
which might be of significance in the patient with cardiac damage.

The material is venous blood, citrated to prevent coagulation.
The blood is inoculated on to blood plates and into broth, and
aerobic and anaerobic culture carried out as in routine bacteriological examination.

Mycological Investigations

By far the most common fungus likely to be encountered in the
oral cavity as a pathogen is Candida albicans (Monilia albicans).
Examination for this organism is best carried out by direct examination of an unstained smear of a scraping from the suspect
area. Under low power magnification the branching mycelia and
blastospores are easily recognisable. Culture of the organisms
may be carried out by growth on glucose agar plates, to confirm
the diagnosis.

In a number of lesions - for example, candidal leukoplakia -
the candidal pseudo-hyphae are within the tissue rather than

superficial to it. In these circumstances they may be recognised
in biopsy tissue on staining with P.A.S. (periodic acid - Schiff)
reagent (Fig. 3.2). It may well be that a heavily infected
lesion of this kind may yield an insignificant growth on superficial swabbing. It should be remembered, when interpreting the
reports on oral flora, that many individuals carry a population
of candida albicans in the oral cavity in a commensal, non-
pathogenic form. It is therefore difficult to assess the significance of light growths of candida on culture.

Agglutination and immunofluorescent tests are available for
application in the study of the immune response of patients with
severe and persistent candidiasis. The methods adopted closely
parallel those used in the case of syphilis. These studies are
not normally carried out in the case of minor degrees of candidiasis.

Very rarely fungal infections involving Histoplasma capsulatum
or Blastomyces dermatitidis may be suspected. Identification may
be carried out, often with difficulty, by examination of biopsy
specimens of the lesions (in which the organisms may be shown up
well in polarized light), by attempts to grow the organisms, and
by the application of a histoplasmin sensitivity test. An immunofluorescent method is also available. Cases of histoplasmosis
and blastomycosis are rare in Europe but of greater frequency in
America and occasionally present with oral lesions.

Investigation of Viral Infections

A number of viral infections involve the oral mucosa.
Although there are characteristic clinical patterns the lesions
produced as a result of differing infections are often so similar
as to be indistinguishable on clinical examination. During the
viral replication which lead to eventual death of the affected
cells there is a complex series of nuclear changes which precede
degeneration. These include the production of intra nuclear
inclusion bodies and, sometimes, cell fusion to form multinucleated cells. These may be detected in epithelial smears from
the lesions and may therefore be taken as reasonable confirmation
of their viral aetiology (Fig. 3.3). They are not, however, any
more specific than this. It need hardly be said that the inclusion bodies represent cellular changes and not the viral particles
themselves which are of a very much smaller order of size.

Positive viral identification may be carried out in several
ways, if the facilities are available.

(1) Antibody titrations. A rise in the serum levels of
    specific antibody during the course of the disease is
    the most precise method of identification of the virus
    involved. Single values are quite useless since
    normal levels vary widely from person to person. It
    is therefore necessary to measure the increase in
    antibody levels in response to the infection. A ten
    day period, starting from the earliest available time
    is usual.

(2)   Culture of virus on fertile egg membranes, in
       animals or in tissue culture. Recognisable
       characteristic lesions may be produced and may
       aid identification by confirming the serological
       results.

(3)   Direct recognition of virions by electron
       microscopic examination of infected tissues
       (Fig. 3.4). This, until recently considered
       a research method, is now coming into much
       more widespread use for routine diagnosis.

(4)   Immunofluorescent tests for antigen in affected
       cells.

It must be stressed, however, that none of these investigations are simple, all are expensive and that the facilities for
them to be carried out are relatively restricted.

Infective Mononucleosis

A serological test used in the detection of infective mononucleosis (glandular fever) is the Paul-Bunnell reaction. In
this, use is made of the observed fact that the serum from a
patient in this condition causes agglutination of sheep red
blood cells. The mechanism of the reaction is not known. The
material for the test is a venous blood sample of some 10 ml. A
screening test is first carried out using the simple agglutination described. If this proves positive, the test is completed
by repeating it with portions of the test sera which have been in
contact with guinea-pig kidney and ox red blood cells. An occasional positively reacting normal serum protein is absorbed by the
guinea-pig cells but not the ox red blood cells, whilst a positive reacting protein occasionally found after injection including
horse serum is absorbed by both. If the screen test is reported
as positive and the completed test as negative then it means that
one of these two possibilities has occurred. If the screen test
is reported negative no further action is taken. If both screen
and completed tests are positive then there is strong evidence
for infective mononucleosis.

Serum Hepatitis (Hepatitis B)

Patients who have had an attack of hepatitis caused by the
type B virus are known to have a residual infective potential.
These high risk patients may be recognised by the presence of a
viral surface antigen (the Australia antigen) in the serum
although the presence of this antigen is not necessarily a mark
of infective potential. Radioimmune assay techniques similar to
those described above are used to detect the presence of this
antigen, the test being very sensitive. In view of the possibly
highly infective nature of the blood under examination specimen
collection must be carried out with great care and specimens
should be transmitted in specially prepared packs with suitable
warning labels.

Chapter IV

Facial Pain

The diagnosis of facial pain can be one of the most perplexing problems facing the dental surgeon. The oral cavity is in close relation to many structures with which it shares common innervations. Pathological changes in the teeth of these associated structures may produce pain symptoms difficult to differentiate.

The matter may be further complicated by the difficulties which may be met by the patient in describing his symptoms accurately. On the whole, however, the terms used by patients to describe pain - "stabbing, throbbing, dull ache" and so on are fairly constant and related to the aetiology of the pain.

The reaction of the patient to pain depends on two factors independent of the strength of the pain stimulus. These are the pain threshold for the patient (the degree of stimulation necessary for the patient to perceive pain) and the individual sensitivity to the pain when perceived. These two factors vary greatly from patient to patient and, in the case of the individual sensitivity, may vary from time to time in the same patient, depending on general health and other transient factors.

When a problem of facial pain arises the greatest efforts must be made to eliminate any possibility of simple dental pathology. In addition to the normal clinical examination of teeth and soft tissues, adequate radiographs of both jaws should be obtained and all teeth tested for vitality and for the presence of sensitive cementum. Only after ruling out all possibility of such relatively simple causes of pain should more complex conditions be sought.

Projected and Referred Pain

If a pain pathway is subjected to stimulation at some point along its course it is possible for pain to be felt in the peripheral distribution of the nerve. This is projected pain. An example of this is the facial pain which may occur in patients with intra cranial neoplasms. The lesion in this case is causing pressure on a central part of the trigeminal pathway, whilst the pain symptoms are felt in the peripheral distribution of the nerve.

This must be distinguished from referred pain in which the pain is felt in an area distant from that in which the causative pathology is located. In the dental field perhaps the most common example of referred pain is that in which pain is felt, for instance, in the maxillary teeth due to a lesion in a mandibular tooth. In this case the pain impulses originate in the

diseased tooth and if the pathway from this tooth is blocked -
say by a local anaesthetic - then the referred pain will cease.
Thus, in our dental example, anaesthesia of the mandibular branch
of the trigeminal nerve will relieve the pain felt in the area
supplied by the maxillary branch. This gives the basis of the
most useful test for the investigation of suspected referred
pain.

    The mechanism of projected pain is fairly clear, but that of
referred pain is by no means so obvious. There is still considerable discussion among investigators as to the true site at
which the "crossover" occurs leading to the sensory misinterpre-
tation of the impulses transmitted from the diseased site.

The Nerve Supply to the Face

    The sensory nerve supply to the face and oral tissues is
shared between a number of nerves - the trigeminal nerve, the
glossopharyngeal nerve and the branches of the cervical plexus.
However, the great majority of pain symptoms in the face are
felt in the area covered by the trigeminal nerve. There is
usually a clear cut distinction between the zones supplied by the
various terminal branches of the trigeminal nerve, with very
little overlap, but there is often considerable overlap between
the trigeminal and cutaneous branches of the cervical plexus
where these are adjacent. Apart from areas of overlap there is
also a complex series of interconnections between the trigeminal,
facial and glossopharyngeal nerves and the nerves arising from
the autonomic nervous system - in particular the sympathetic
fibres associated with blood vessels severing the area. These
sympathetic fibres may play some part in the transmission of
deep impulses - it has been shown that such pain can be produced by the stimulation of the superior cervical sympathetic
ganglion. Similarly, it has been shown that pain impulses from
the deeper facial structures may be transmitted by the proprio-
ceptive fibres of the facial nerve. However, there is little
agreement among the various workers who have investigated these
secondary pain pathways as to their clinical significance.

Facial Pain

    The great majority of patients complaining of pain in and
about the face are suffering from some form of toothache.
However, there are many other possible causes of such pain.
The structures related to the mouth which might give rise to
pain symptoms are so complex and the innervation of these structures so interrelated that errors in diagnosis are easily made.
The main sensory nerve of the area - the trigeminal nerve -
eventually divides into a large number of small terminal branches supplying the skin of a large part of the face and scalp as
well as the majority of the oral tissues and many deeper structures. Although the superficial limits of the trigeminal nerve
can be accurately determined with little overlap the deeper
limits are much less well defined and understood. It is often
difficult to determine the point at which a facial pain becomes
a headache and there may be consequent difficulties in communic-
ation between the patient and the investigator.

It is convenient to consider facial pain as being of four
types:-

    1.   Pain resulting from recognisable pathological
change in the oral, facial and closely associated
structures. Examples are toothache, the pain of
maxillary sinusitis and pain associated with
temporo-mandibular joint disturbance.

    2.   Pain of unknown origin felt in the face. This
includes trigeminal neuralgia and the so-called
"atypical facial pain" - a mysterious but very
troublesome condition which will be discussed
later.

    3.   Pain projected to the face due to pathological
change affecting the pain pathways central to
the facial structures. Secondary neuralgia
caused by pressure of a neoplasm on the trigeminal
nerve is a rare example of this group. Migraine
(not strictly a facial pain) could also be
classified in this way because of its aetiology -
changes in the intracranial blood vessels.

    4.   Pain referred to the face from distant areas of
the body. An example of this are in angina
pectoris, in which pain may be felt over the
left mandible.

It should be stressed that there is no characteristic pattern
of pain associated with any of these four groups. They form only
an arbitrary series of headings under which facial pain may be
considered when presenting for diagnosis and, in the subsequent
discussions there will be seen to be a number of factors which
must be regarded as common between the groups.

The Investigation of Facial Pain

The objective investigation of pain is extremely difficult.
Pain in itself produces no detectable signs and the basis of the
whole investigation is the description given by the patient. This
may be so coloured by a variety of personal factors as to be con-
fusing and misleading. All pain causes a mental reaction and it
is often impossible to differentiate between "normal" and
"abnormal" reactions because of a complete lack of any means of
objective measurement of the intensity of the pain. The function
of pain in giving an early warning of pathological changes is
notoriously erratic, and the excessive degree of pain associated
with many conditions seems quite disproportionate if regarded as a
warning sign. Many of the clinical conditions seen by the dental
surgeon seem to fall into this category in which minor (or even
quite unrecognisable) pathological changes elicit a quite disproportionate response leading to great distress in the individual
concerned.

The investigation of a patient complaining of facial pain is
carried out in two stages. In the first stage an assessment of

the pain is made relative to the dental apparatus (teeth and
supporting tissues) and the closely related structures such as
the maxillary antra and the temporo-mandibular joints - this
corresponding to the first group defined above. If, after full
examination, no abnormalities are found in these areas the
investigator is justified in considering other possibilities. If
the essential first step of eliminating dental causes of the pain
is omitted confusion is bound to follow in many cases.

Pain of Local Origin

Dental Pain
     The first step in the investigation of the patient with facial
pain is to eliminate the possibility of toothache or pain of
periodontal origin. This may be less easy than it first appears.
The classic methods of assessment by probe and mirror reinforced
by thermal or electrical stimulation of the teeth, percussion
mobility testing and radiography, although the essential basis
of the examination may not always be relied on to give an accurate result. Particularly in the case of heavily filled teeth
there should be no hesitation in removing the restoration in
order to get a better indication of tooth vitality or to confirm
hypersensitivity. It should be remembered that it can be by no
means certain whether a non vital tooth is or is not a source of
pain but valuable evidence may be got in this way. Local anaesthesia may be invaluable in helping to localise the pain to a
tooth (or group of teeth) by temporarily abolishing the pain
symptoms, and indeed this is a useful technique in the investigation of the source of facial pain of all kinds.

     The complexity of this subject, which for long has been
considered to be a quite straightforward one, may be judged by
the fact that Mumford (1973) is able to devote six chapters of a
substantial book to the diagnosis of toothache arising from
varying sources. Without a discussion of this depth it must be
stressed that no investigation of facial pain should omit the
essential first step - the elimination of dental causes. The
list of specific factors to be eliminated is long but includes
(as some of the more obvious):-

                    Caries (primary and recurrent)
                    Pulps of abnormal vitality reaction
                    Inadequately lined, fractured or leaking
                    fillings.
                    Fractured or cracked teeth.
                    Traumatic occlusion - including "high" fillings.
                    Root filled teeth.
                    Exposed dentine or cementum.
                    Impacted teeth.
                    Teeth with periapical or periodontal lesions.
                    Buried teeth, roots or apices.

     The nature of the pain arising from causes such as these is
by no means specific and no particular factor should be ignored
on the basis of an uncharacteristic pain. The relationship

between acute and chronic pulpitis and definite pain patterns,
long accepted, has now been clearly shown to be totally erratic
and indeed, the clinical usage of these terms is quite unrelated
to the cellular changes actually occurring in the affected pulps.

Pain of Temporo-Mandibular Joint Origin

The symptoms of temporo-mandibular joint disturbance and the
pain arising from this condition are discussed in Chapter VIII.
It should be remembered that pain of temporo-mandibular joint
origin may be widely distributed and may simulate the symptoms of
a wide range of conditions. In any investigation of facial pain
of unknown origin, however unusual the symptoms, the possibility
of joint disturbance and consequential pain should always be kept
in mind.

In general there are physical signs of some kind - either
primary or secondary - which give a lead to the possible diagnosis
of pain of joint origin. Although the more obvious, such as
joint clicks, occlusal irregularities or tenderness over the
condyles may be missing in some cases, there are few patients
with pain of joint origin who, after careful examination, do not
show at least some of the signs discussed in Chapter VIII.

Maxillary Sinusitis

The nature of the pain arising from maxillary sinusitis
depends largely on whether the infection is acute or chronic. In
acute sinusitis the pain is often intense and is located in and
around the affected sinus. Nearby structures are often involved
and there may be swelling of the face in the infra-orbital area.
Similarly, nearby teeth may become sensitive and tender to percussion. There is often a bloodstained nasal discharge and the
patient suffers considerable malaise. In chronic sinusitis the
pain is usually less severe and is generally described as being a
dull ache. Again it is often localised in the area of the affected sinus but there may be referred pain to the frontal or temporal area and again the teeth may be affected and become tender
to percussion. There may be variation in the pain according to
the posture of the patient depending on the level of the fluid
exudate within the affected sinus. X-ray usually shows a thick-
ened lining to the affected sinuses together with the presence of
fluid. However, in early acute sinusitis there may be little
radiographic change, even though the symptoms may be severe.

The symptoms of maxillary sinusitis, both acute and chronic,
are easily mistaken for those arising from a dental abscess.
Indeed, there may be a close association as in the case of oro-
antral fistulae or periapical infections spreading from the maxillary teeth into the antrum.

Facial Pain of Unknown Origin

Neuralgia

The definition of neuralgia depends on a number of rather
diffuse clinical factors. It is perhaps best thought of as a
pain localised to an area supplied by a single sensory nerve,
paroxysmal and severe in nature. A number of conditions give

rise to pain of this nature in and about the face. Many classifications are possible but the most important distinction is between primary and secondary neuralgias. Primary neuralgia
implies a condition in which the pain is present without any
known initiating pathology. This does not mean to imply that
pathological change does not occur - simply that none has as yet
been detected. The most common primary neuralgia is that affecting the trigeminal nerve in one or more of its sensory branches,
but a very similar although less common condition affects the
glossopharyngeal nerve. In secondary neuralgias precisely similar pain may occur, but pathological changes affecting the
course of the involved nerve can be recognised. This pathological change may affect any part of the nerve, from the periphery
to the central sensory nuclei, the pain being projected to the
peripheral distribution. Thus in the case of the trigeminal
nerve secondary facial neuralgias may occur as the result of
neoplasia, trauma or inflammatory change affecting the extra or
intra cranial course of the nerve.

It should be pointed out that various clinical conditions
occasionally arise in which pain similar to that described may
occur, but which is not usually considered to be a neuralgia.
For instance, pain of temporo-mandibular joint origin may occasionally simulate that of a neuralgia. Some authorities would
consider this to be a secondary trigeminal neuralgia, but it is
perhaps better to reserve this term for those conditions in which
an extraneous pathological process impinges upon the sensory
pathways of the trigeminal nerve.

Trigeminal Neuralgia
Trigeminal neuralgia is a disease of such characteristic
intensity that it has been known and described over a long period
of history. In spite of this, the true nature of this extremely
painful condition is not known. Although pain is normally considered to be a symptom rather than a disease, the lack of other
associated symptoms and of basic knowledge as to aetiology makes
it at present necessary to consider the pain as being the disease itself. Numerous investigations into the nature of the
disease have been carried out in recent years but, probably due
to the extreme difficulty in obtaining material for histological
or ultrastructural investigation, these have as yet proved
fruitless.

Trigeminal neuralgia is, in general, a disease of patients of
more than middle age, some 70% being over the age of 50 years
before the first symptoms appear. Should pain of this kind
occur in a younger patient, it is often the first symptom of a
generalised neurological disturbance - usually disseminated
sclerosis. The characteristic feature of the disease is intense
pain in one side of the face. For some reason the right side of
the face is affected more often than the left. Bilateral cases
are, fortunately, extremely rare. The pain is most often localised to one of the branches of the trigeminal nerve, at least in
the early stages, but there are cases in which two or three
branches of the nerve are involved from the beginning. The pain
is characteristically excruciatingly severe, of rapid onset and

of short duration. It is usually described by the patient as a
series of shooting or stabbing pains. It is generally accepted
that between the attacks of pain, which may last for no more
than a few seconds, there is no other pain felt. The periods
between attacks may vary between a few minutes to several hours.
The presence of a trigger zone is a feature of the disease in
many patients (but not all). This is an area, either on the
face or the oral mucosa, on which the slightest touch appears to
stimulate an attack of the pain. The trigger zone may or may not
be within the area of distribution of the pain. In the presence
of such a trigger zone the patient finds it difficult to wash the
face or to shave and in some cases the sensitivity of the zone is
such that the movement of the air is sufficient to precipitate an
attack. This accounts for the "frozen face" exhibited by many
patients. In virtually all cases the pain is restricted to the
daytime - the patients are not wakened by the pain at night.

In the very early stages of the disease there may be a period
in which the pain is non-characteristic. It is at this time that
the patients are most often seen by the dental surgeon for the
investigation of what may be highly perplexing pain symptoms. It
is also at this stage of the disease that the patient may ascribe
the pain to toothache in what may appear to be an entirely sound
tooth. Following the extraction of this tooth the pain may then
be described as coming from a nearby tooth and extraction of this
may also be demanded by the patient. It is not rare to find
patients made virtually unilaterally edentulous in this way. Many
eventual difficulties can be avoided if it is recognised that any
patient presenting with this pattern of symptoms should be considered as worthy of full investigation before further extractions
are considered.

Conversely the situation may arise in which pain closely resembling trigeminal neuralgia may arise from some quite ordinary
dental pathology such as a retained root or an unerupted tooth or
even from unsatisfactory dentures. If there is any abnormality
of this kind present it should be treated as the essential first
step in the management of the patient.

Local anaesthetic injections may be of value in accurately
localising the involved nerve branch, and it is often found to be
the case that, following the period of anaesthesia, there is an
interval during which further attacks of pain do not occur. However, within a day or two at the most the pain is found to return
unchanged. If a trigger zone is present it is possible to inactivate it by a very small amount of local anaesthetic in the area.
If the zone is on the oral mucosa, a local anaesthetic paste or
solution applied superficially is often sufficient to inactivate
the triggering mechanism. It should be stressed that it is the
trigger area to which the anaesthetic is applied - not the area
of the pain symptoms. Drug therapy of trigeminal neuralgia
depends almost entirely on its variable response to carbamazepine
(Tegretol). A positive response to therapy of this kind is a
strong confirmatory support of the clinical diagnosis. The reverse is not so, since some patients do not respond.

Glossopharyngeal Neuralgia

Glossopharyngeal neuralgia is a similar condition to that of the trigeminal nerve, but much less common. The pain is of the same nature as that in trigeminal neuralgia and is unilaterally felt in the oropharynx, sometimes with pain referred to the ear. Although the main component of the pain is described (as in trigeminal neuralgia) as stabbing or shooting in nature, there may also be an appreciable residual ache which may last for some time after the paroxysmal attack. The pain is often precipitated by swallowing, and there may be a trigger zone. If such a zone is present, relief of the pain may be achieved by spraying the area with local anaesthetic solution. Treatment with Carbamazepine is successful in the majority of cases and confirms the diagnosis.

Atypical Facial Pain

Among patients presenting with facial pain there is a significant proportion in whom the symptoms seem to be unrelated either to the anatomy of the part involved or to any known pathological process. These are the patients who are described as having atypical facial pain. This is a diagnostic term which is vague and unsatisfactory and which is used to describe a wide spectrum of symptoms, but for the particular patients described no better diagnostic grouping has as yet been suggested.

The characteristics of the patients involved can be summarised:-

(1) The facial pain is not necessarily described as being confined to the trigeminal area or to any other anatomically distinct area. The pain may be said to spread over an extremely wide area, occasionally to the upper and lower limbs.

(2) The pain may be bilateral. In assessing this factor it should be remembered, however, that by far the commonest condition in which bilateral facial pain occurs is temporomandibular joint dysfunction.

(3) The pain is usually described as being constant and, often, as lasting over a very long period of time. A description of a pain lasting constantly, night and day, over many years, is not uncommon. The nature of the pain is usually described as being a severe ache felt in deep as well as in more superficial structures.

(4) The patient may be suffering from some quite evident psychiatric disturbance. However this is by no means so in every case. In those patients who are evidently disturbed the description of the pain may be bizarre and such a patient may spend a high proportion of his life moving between practitioners of various

disciplines in order to gain further
opinions on his symptoms.

There is little uniformity between the patients involved, the
only common linking factors being that all investigations prove
negative and that all attempts at treatment make matters worse
rather than better.

Pain of Central Origin Projected to the Face

Migraine

Migraine presents essentially as a headache but there is sometimes associated facial pain and the patient may well be seen for
elimination of a dental cause for his symptoms. The predominating symptom is an intense periodic headache. This is usually
unilateral, but may occasionally be bilateral and may spread into
the face. The pain is felt in the anterior temporal region and
its facial extension is over the maxilla. In a few cases the
pain may extend downwards into the neck. The pain lasts for a
period of some hours or even, in protracted attacks, for several
days. A number of other neurological disturbances may be associated with the headache, the most common being nausea, vomiting
and visual disturbances. The subject suffers from considerable
malaise during an attack and frequently needs bed rest until the
symptoms subside. Migraine and its variants often occur in members of a family - an important point in history taking.

The basic cause of this condition appears to be vasodilation
of the cranial arteries. Many of the patients suffering from
migraine are under some degree of mental stress, often occupying
positions of responsibility under conditions of tension. It
seems also that certain foods - for instance chocolate - may
initiate an attack in susceptible individuals.

Acute Migrainous Neuralgia (Cluster Headache)

This condition is similar in aetiology to migraine but with a
different clinical presentation. The patient suffers from periodic attacks of severe pain lasting in most cases about thirty
minutes, unilateral and located behind the eye, with occasional
spread to the temporal region and to the maxilla. Unusually
among the facial pains of non-dental origin the attacks often
occur at night. There is usually irritation and lachrymation of
the eye on the affected side and, often, blocking of the nostril.
The attacks are closely concentrated over a period of one or two
days and nights. The patient is then free of attacks for a period often of several weeks. This 'clustering' of the attacks
leads to one of the many alternative names for this condition.
Two other names still used are Horton's syndrome and histamine
cephalgia. The patients are predominantly male (80%) and the
condition begins at an early age (between 17 and 25 years in more
than 50% of cases). The patients occasionally present for investigation as possible cases of pain of dental origin, particularly
when the maxilla is involved in the painful area. The diagnosis
depends entirely on the characteristic history.

Facial Pain in Herpes Zoster

The pain associated with herpes zoster is probably best considered as a pain of central origin projected to the face, since the essential lesion is a viral neuritis affecting not only a peripheral branch or branches of the trigeminal nerve but also the ganglion itself. Of the peripheral branches of the nerve the first is the most often affected.

The pain may be present for a few days before the appearance of the skin eruption. It is usually described as a severe stinging or burning pain but occasionally paroxysmal pain may occur, similar to that of trigeminal neuralgia. Two or three days after the onset of the pain the characteristic herpetic vesicles appear on the skin of the affected area. These may last from one to two weeks before slowly fading. In most cases the pain disappears shortly after the resolution of the vesicles. In a few patients, however, the pain may persist for a much longer time - sometimes for years, occasionally permanently. Occasionally also the pain, once having disappeared with the fading of the vesicles, may return after quite a long pain free period.

The diagnosis of this pain may prove difficult in the prevesicular phase, although there is often a considerable degree of malaise which, together with the distribution of the pain, may help to give an indication of its origin. Post herpetic pain is usually at its most severe and protracted in older patients and is highly resistant to all forms of treatment.

Pain from Neoplasms and Nerve Compression

Facial pain and headache may be symptoms of a wide variety of intra and extra cranial lesions such as neoplasms or vascular abnormalities. Facial pain may arise by involvement (either by pressure or by malignant infiltration of the trigeminal ganglion of the peripheral branches of the nerve. Primary and secondary intra cranial neoplasms, nasopharyngeal tumours, aneurysms and cerebral epidermoid cysts are among the most commonly recorded of lesions of this type causing facial pain. Similarly the lesions left following brain damage of any kind may be the source of facial pain. In cases of this type facial pain is only rarely the only symptom, although it may well be the earliest. Involvement of other cranial nerves and the presence of unusual symptoms such as anaesthesia or paraesthesia should at once raise the suspicion of the possibility of a lesion of this kind.

Another cause of facial pain arising from compression of the trigeminal nerve is in Paget's disease affecting the base of the skull. Some degree of closure of the foramina is common and the consequent stricture of the nerve may lead to a variety of pain symptoms. A further cause of trauma to the trigeminal nerve in Paget's disease may be the deformation of the skull as a whole causing compression of the sensory root of the nerve where it crosses the petrous bone. The pain often simulates trigeminal neuralgia, although aching pains may be sometimes reported.

A similar compression of the auditory nerve may give rise to
deafness and changes in the cervical spine may also lead to pain
in the area served by the sensory nerves of the cervical plexus.

A more peripheral form of nerve compression leading to pain
may be seen in post traumatic fibrosis around the infra-orbital
foramen following fracture of the anterior wall of the maxillary
sinus with involvement of the foramen. This line of fracture is
common in injuries to the maxillo-zygomatic complex. Very occasionally, a similar fibrosis may follow infection in the area -
say following a periapical infection on a maxillary canine tooth.
The pain produced is usually paroxysmal, but not of the severe
nature of trigeminal neuralgia. It is certainly wise, if trigeminal neuralgia confined to the infra-orbital nerve is suspected, to consider the possibility of such a fibrous stricture.

Pain Referred to the Face from Distant Areas

Perhaps the most significant pain of this nature is that
which may be felt over the left mandible in cases of coronary
insufficiency. This is usually no more than the accompaniment
to other and more characteristic pain - retrosternal pain radiating down the left arm in many cases. However, a few cases have
been reported in which the pain in the face was the only symptom
recorded before an episode of myocardial infarction. It follows
that a cardiac origin must be considered as a possible diagnosis
if unexplained pain is present in this location.

A few cases of referral of pain originating in far distant
structures have been reported, but these are so sparse in number
that they have little more than curiosity interest. However, it
is worth recalling that the patient with psychogenic facial pain
may produce a multiplicity of widespread symptoms which lead to
great difficulties in diagnosis if the true nature of the condition is not recognised.

Temporal Headache
Two conditions which may very occasionally be seen by the
dental surgeon - although not strictly facial pains - are temporal arteritis and the auriculo-temporal syndrome (Frey's syndrome).

In temporal arteritis the pain is localised to the temporal
and frontal regions - the area supplied by the superficial temporal artery. The pain is described as a severe ache, but paroxysmal pain is occasionally also described. In between attacks
of pain the affected area may be very tender to the touch. The
patients, most of whom are in older age groups, also complain of
general malaise and diffuse muscular and joint pains. There may
also be degeneration of vision. The essential pathology of this
condition is a generalised inflammatory lesion of the arteries
which shows itself early in the superficial temporal artery.

The auriculo temporal syndrome is caused by irritation of the
auriculo temporal nerve as it passes through the substance of the

parotid gland in the early part of its course. The irritation
may be the result of a wide range of pathological processes
within the gland, both inflammatory and neoplastic or by surgical
trauma. The symptoms are of pain in the distribution of the
auriculo temporal nerve, usually described as burning in nature,
and associated with excessive sweating and erythema in the area
during eating. Between attacks of pain there may be anaesthesia
or paraesthesia of the skin in the affected area. It is evident
that, the condition being recognised, confirmation of the diagnosis and subsequent treatment depends on a full investigation
of the involved parotid gland.

Anaesthesia and Paraesthesia

The onset of anaesthesia or paraesthesia, either slowly or
suddenly, in the distribution of a nerve is a sign of a lesion
at some point along the nerve path. If such a condition occurs,
the following oral and dental causes must be eliminated before
more central or systemic disturbances are sought:-

Fracture of the jaw, involving the nerve canal.
Severance of the nerve in oral surgery.
Pressure on the nerve by a foreign body (e.g. tooth
root in canal).
Transient trauma during operation or following an
injection.
Inflammatory changes (especially osteomyelitis) in
relation to the nerve.
Neoplasia encroaching on the nerve.

If no such peripheral cause for the condition is found then
neurological investigation is indicated.

Chapter V

Lesions of the Teeth and Periodontium

The teeth are poor indicators of generalised disease. Following their calcification metabolic processes have little effect on the structure of the teeth and the only major changes which ordinarily occur are the loss of substance caused by caries, attrition, erosion and abrasion. Other structural abnormalities almost invariably reflect changes occurring in the period during which the teeth were being formed. Apart from structural variation, abnormalities in the numbers, size and shape of the teeth occasionally occur in conjunction with abnormalities of the bones or of the skin and other epidermally derived structures. When numbers of missing teeth, supernumerary teeth or abnormally shaped teeth are observed it is as well to consider the possibility of some such complex association. It must always be remembered that teeth missing from the arch may be either congenitally absent, have been extracted or may be unerupted. The presence of unerupted teeth is detected by the taking of adequate radiographs of the area in question.

Partial Anodontia

Partial anodontia represented by the loss of one or two teeth with no apparent associated abnormalities is not uncommon. World wide studies show that the teeth thus missing vary from population to population. A study carried out in an English population and excluding the third molars has shown that the teeth most likely to be missing are the lower second premolars (40.9%) followed by the upper lateral incisors (23.5%) and by the upper second premolars (20.9%). Other teeth are much less frequently missing. In the case of the upper lateral incisor it has been shown in several populations that the absence of this tooth (or teeth - the loss is often bilateral) is genetically determined. The third molars also show a wide variation in the pattern of absence determined in differing populations. Most surveys however, show that one or more third molars are missing in approximately one quarter of the population.

A characteristic finding in partial anodontia is the presence of small and conically shaped teeth replacing normal units of the dentition (Fig. 5.1). These simple structures represent a single cusp rather than the fused series of cusps which together form the normal tooth. It appears that these simple teeth represent a half way stage to total suppression. It is not uncommon, for example, for one upper lateral incisor to be completely lost whilst the opposite tooth is found to be of the conical type.

There has been little work carried out on partial anodontia

in the primary dentition but it would seem that this is a relatively rare occurrence. It does seem, however, that from time to
time the same tooth may be missing from the deciduous and from
the permanent dentition.

Partial anodontia associated with abnormalities of the bone or
ectodermal appendages is relatively rare. The dysplasia involved
may be attributed to ectodermally derived structures (as in anhi-
drotic ectodermal dysplasia Fig. 5.2) or with more complex syndromes (such as the Hallerman-Strieff syndrome Fig. 5.3) in which
there are both dermal and bony abnormalities.

Supernumerary teeth may occur at almost any point in the
dental arch and are usually of little other significance. It
must be remembered however that a frequent consequence of the
presence of the supernumerary teeth in the anterior region of
the maxilla is a failure of the normal teeth to erupt. Thus the
most common sign of the presence of such supernumerary teeth is
the absence of a permanent incisor from the arch. Patients with
cleft palates are fairly frequently found to have supernumerary
teeth. These are most often of the small conical type and
closely associated with the margins of the cleft.

The only more widespread condition in which the presence of
many supernumerary teeth is common is cleido-cranial dysostosis.
In this abnormality of membrane bone formation the changes observed are lack of calcification of the clavicle, flattening of
the frontal bone and the presence of a number of supernumerary
teeth. These teeth are often of complex form, resembling units
of the normal dentition, and frequently remain unerupted (Fig.
5.4). A parodoxical feature of this condition is that it may
appear that the patient is suffering from partial anodontia
because of the failure to erupt of large numbers of teeth within
the jaws. It is often quite impossible to distinguish the teeth
of the normal dentition from those of the abnormal dentition.
The presence of such numbers of unerupted teeth of mature form is
quite characteristic of cleido-cranial dysostosis and should be
followed up by the taking of confirmatory radiographs of the
skull and clavicles.

Variation in Dates of Eruption of the Teeth
    The wide normal range makes it difficult to specify accurately
the dates of eruption of either the deciduous or the permanent
teeth. A number of factors has been found to affect the date of
eruption, including racial origin and such unlikely influences as
the socio-economic environment. In general, earlier bodily development is reflected in early eruption of the teeth.

Markedly premature eruption of the permanent teeth is very
rare. It has been suggested that it may occur in cases of hyper-
secretion of those hormones which influence development. It is
somewhat more common to note premature eruption of the deciduous
teeth. Frequently no systemic factor is found to account for
this. It should perhaps be mentioned that teeth present at birth
in a few children (the neo-natal teeth) do not represent premature eruption. These are supernumerary teeth and part of a

separate pre-deciduous dentition.

Delayed eruption of the deciduous teeth may occur in endocrine deficiency states and it has been shown that in Down's syndrome (mongolism) not only are the eruption dates somewhat retarded in general but also there is often an unusual sequence of eruption. It is very difficult to ascribe a characteristic dental picture to many of the endocrine abnormalities since, in a number of cases, varying and contradictory effects have been described. In many such patients the most obvious abnormality is disproportion in the sizes of the teeth and the jaws, this in turn leading to gross irregularity of the occlusion.

Variation in the Size of Teeth
The size of the teeth of any individual is determined largely by inherited factors. Extreme variation in size, either in the direction of small teeth (microdontism) or in the direction of large teeth (macrodontism) may be accompanied by no other growth abnormality. Conversely, endocrine growth disorders leading to gigantism or dwarfism may be accompanied by no corresponding variation in tooth size. A few cases of hemifacial gigantism have, however, been recorded in which unilateral macrodontia has occurred.

It follows that the size of the teeth alone bears no relationship to metabolic factors in the vast majority of instances and that diagnostic significance cannot be given to such variation, excepting as an observed developmental factor.

Variation in Cusp and Root Form of Teeth
Variation in cusp form of the teeth usually extends to the suppression or exaggeration of the normally present cusps, although extra cusps may be present. These extra cusps probably represent an adventitious extra fold in the enamel organ with no other significance. Similarly the presence of extra roots has little other than local significance, although the presence of bilateral extra roots, as frequently occurs, suggests rather more than a random accidental splitting of Hertwig's sheath during root formation.

Occasionally the variation in tooth form may be so great as to be regarded as more than a simple aberration of cusp or root development. In these cases the tooth may be regarded as an odontome. Of these the most common form is the invaginated odontome in which an infolding of the enamel epithelium during development has produced an effect varying from a small depression on the cingulum to a large dilatation within the tooth (Fig. 5.5).

The more considerably affected of these odontomes may be readily diagnosed by appearance and by radiographic evidence. The simpler forms, however (a of Fig. 5.5), may be distinguished only by a very small pit on the cingulum of an anterior tooth. The pit may, however, be deep and pass well into the proximity of the pulp chamber. Caries in the depths of such a deep invagination may lead to the death of the tooth. Occasionally dilatation of the root may occur with relatively normal crown form.

Invaginated odontomes in the anterior region are frequently bilateral and should be suspected and carefully looked for in the case of otherwise inexplicable pulp death, particularly in young patients.

Gemination (the fusion of two teeth) may occur in two ways. Pathological gemination is the joining together of teeth by excess secondary cementum formed in response to chronic inflammatory changes in the periodontal tissues. Diagnosis of this may occasionally be made radiographically but is all too often made only when there is an attempt to extract one of the joined pair. The condition is most frequently seen in the case of the maxillary second and unerupted third molars.

Physiological or true gemination occurs as a result of the fusion of two tooth germs during development. This may occur either between the germs of two normally adjacent teeth, or between the resultant halves of a germ which has been divided by some fault in development. Some authorities use the term 'fusion' for the first of these alternatives and restrict the term 'germination' to the second. The junction tissue between the two components of the geminated pair may be either dentine or enamel, and there may be either a single or double root canal depending on the stage of tooth germ development at which the split occurred. The condition is not usually bilateral.

Erosion

Erosion has been defined by Pindborg as the loss of dental hard tissue by a chemical process which does not involve bacteria. The active substance may be acid spray (as in the metal finishing industries), medicines of low pH or acidic foodstuffs and beverages. Occasionally acid regurgitation may be the cause of the tooth loss. Table V lists a number of the most commonly implicated substances.

TABLE V

BEVERAGES & FOODSTUFFS WHICH MAY CAUSE EROSION

Lemons and juice (fresh, tinned or bottled)
Oranges and juice (fresh, tinned or bottled)
Grapefruit and juice (fresh, tinned or bottled)
Fruit squashes and cordials
Cola type drinks
'Mixer' type drinks (e.g. lemonade, bitter lemon)
Vinegar
Pickled onions
Acidiculated sweets
Ice lollipops

This is evidently an incomplete list but includes the more common offenders.

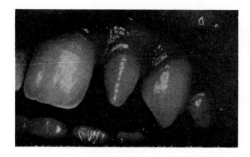 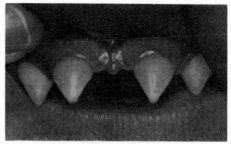

Fig. 5.1   Fig. 5.2

Fig. 5.1. A conically shaped tooth in the position of an upper lateral incisor.
Fig. 5.2. Multiple conical teeth associated
with partial anodontia in anhydriotic ectodermal
dysplasia.

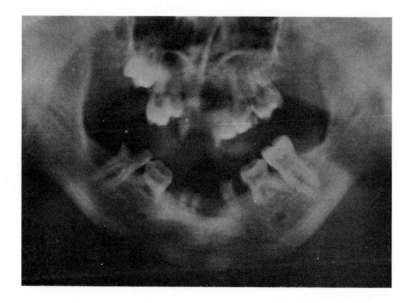

Fig. 5.3. Partial anodontia in the Hallermann-
Strief syndrome. The teeth shown represent the
whole of the adult dentition.

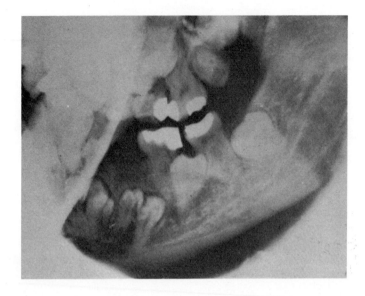

Fig. 5.4. Radiograph of mandible in cleido-
cranial dysostosis, showing multiple unerupted
teeth.

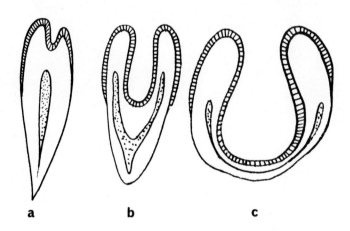

a   b   c

Fig. 5.5. Diagram illustrating various degrees
of invagination. a) represents a simple cingulum
pit, b) and c) represent more advanced degrees
of invagination.

The criteria for diagnosis of erosion are not so clear cut as might be expected since there is often an extra element of abrasion involved. However, it has been suggested (by Eccles & Jenkins) that the criteria should be as follows:-

   1.   Absence of surface detail of the enamel
        resulting in a smooth glazed surface.
        In severe cases there may be complete
        loss of enamel.

   2.   Cavities in the cervical or lingual
        enamel surfaces, distinguished from the
        lesions of abrasion by their shallowness.

   3.   Edges of fillings raised above the level
        of the tooth surface.

   4.   Depressions of the incisal edges of the
        anterior teeth or on the cusps of the
        posterior teeth.

It is pointed out by these authors that abrasion often plays a part in erosion and that the glazed surface of the teeth is in fact due to a polishing rather than to the initial action of the acid. Early and advanced examples of erosion are shown in Figs. 5.6, 5.7.

Abrasion
Abrasion, the loss of tooth substance by mechanical contact with foreign bodies, is most regularly seen in the form of toothbrush abrasion. In such cases the wear is maximal at the gingival margins of the teeth, being particularly pronounced in the canine areas where maximum friction is exerted (Fig. 5.8). It is frequently substantially unilateral, being most marked on the left side in the case of a right-handed patient. The abrasion may be very marked and deep saucer-shaped depressions may be worn from the cervical areas of the teeth, often without any pain symptoms and practically always free from carious attack. Abrasion may occur as a result of wear produced by foreign bodies other than a toothbrush, an example being the groove worn in a maxillary incisor by the frequent use of the tooth to open a hair-grip.

Attrition
Attrition is the loss of tooth substance as a result of interdental wear. It occurs primarily on occluding surfaces and also, to a minor degree, on proximal areas of contact as a result of movement of the teeth during mastication (Fig. 5.9). In the patient eating a refined diet the degree of occlusal attrition is minimal and normally does not lead to exposure of the dentine. Undue attrition in such a patient is usually an indication of occlusal disharmony, particularly in the case of assymetric or unilaterally incomplete dentitions. When the diet is less

refined occlusal attrition is more marked and exposure of the
dentine may be accounted as normal.

Stains and Deposits on Teeth

Extrinsic staining and deposition on the teeth may occur under
many varying circumstances, of which a poor oral hygiene is probably the most common factor. These stains may be differentiated
from intrinsic colorations of the teeth by the relative ease of
their removal by prophylaxis paste and brush.

The colours, types, sites and causative agents for some of
these stains are summarized in Table VI.

TABLE VI

STAINS AND DEPOSITS ON TEETH

Colour	Site on tooth	Causative agent
White (materia alba)	Cervical areas	Poor oral hygiene
Green	Labial surfaces in children	Bacterial - poor oral hygiene
Black	(a) Labial gingival line (a normal finding in many patients)	Not known
	(b) Diffusely over crown	Iron-containing medicines
Brown	(a) Diffusely over crown	Plaque like substances Chlorhexidine
	(b) Lingual, palatal and interproximal areas	Tobacco stain

Intrinsic Staining of Teeth

The most common cause of the discoloration of a single tooth
is the presence in the dentine of decomposition products of
haemoglobin. These find their way into the dentinal tubules
following trauma to the pulp and liberation of haemoglobin from
the erythrocytes. Combination of the breakdown products of the
haemoglobin with those of the associated proteins produces a
range of final products with a wide spectrum of colours ranging
from orange-red to grey, brown and black. Thus a traumatized
tooth may take on a colour depending on the precise nature of

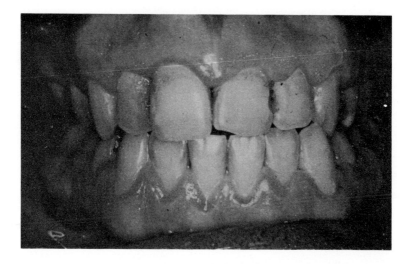

Fig. 5.6. Early erosion. Lesions are seen at the cervical margins of the teeth whilst there is some loss of contour of the surface enamel.

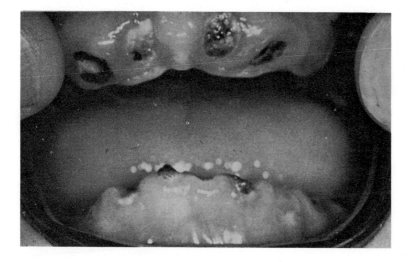

Fig. 5.7. Gross loss of tooth substance initiated by acid erosion. In this extreme case erosion, abrasion and caries have all taken part in the destruction of tissue.

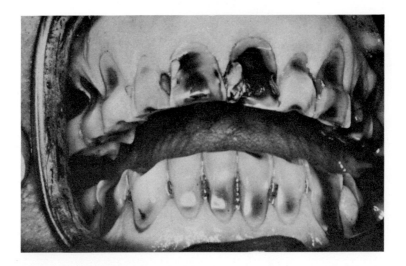

Fig. 5.8. Marked toothbrush abrasion. The
labial enamel is almost completely lost from
many of the teeth.

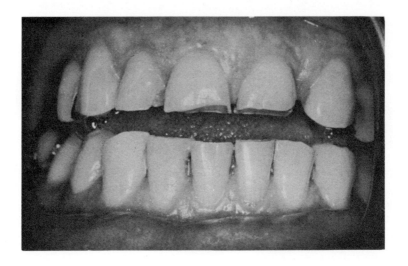

Fig. 5.9. Attrition affecting the incisal surface of the anterior teeth, the result of occlusal disharmony.

these products. Discoloration of this nature does not necessarily imply loss of pulp vitality. It is quite possible for a
pulp to recover from such an incident and to exhibit vitality
when tested.

Staining of a single tooth may also occur by the use of some
materials used in conservative dentistry. Of these silver nit-
rate, which produces a dark grey coloration, is the most common.
Occasionally a copper amalgam restoration may produce the same
effect.

Occasionally a single tooth may be discolored as a result of
idiopathic resorption. In this condition the resorptive facul-
ties of the pulp or of the periodontal membrane are in some
unknown way stimulated to a pathological degree. This may occur
in any tooth, but more commonly in the permanent anterior teeth.
As a result of this abnormal activity an area of dentine is
resorbed and may be replaced by a loose structure of granulation
tissue and by areas of calcified tissue resembling immature bone.
The condition is referred to as external idiopathic resorption if
initiated in periodontal tissue, as internal idiopathic resorption if initiated in pulp.

The process is quite painless unless secondary infection
occurs and is associated with decreased vitality of the pulp to
testing. The condition is often referred to as pink spot and
this well describes the clinical appearance in an advanced case.
Radiographs confirm the presence of the rounded resorbed area in
the pulp chamber which gives the appearance of the pink spot.
Many aetiological features have been suggested, mostly including
trauma in some form. However, it does seem that in some instances the resorption is truly idiopathic although this is difficult
to prove.

Widespread coloration of the teeth occurs in a few diseases in
which abnormal blood pigments circulate. Of these infantile
jaundice is the most common. In this condition the deciduous
teeth may be coloured blue-green due to the laying down of a pig-
ment in the immediate postnatal dentine zone. A less common and
now virtually eliminated cause of tooth discoloration is haemolytic anaemia of the newborn caused by Rh incompatibility. Following the haemolysis pigments may be deposited in the skin and in
the teeth which may take on coloration which varies from grey to
green/grey and to brown. Coloration of the teeth also occurs in
some other considerably rarer situations in which abnormal pigments circulate - for example, in porphyria. However, a far more
common cause of tooth discoloration is tetracycline staining.

Discoloration of the teeth occurs in a high proportion of
children undergoing antibiotic therapy with drugs of the tetracycline group during the time of tooth development. Staining
may also occur as a result of the passing of tetracyclines
through the placenta in the prenatal period. The staining is
grey-brown with chlortetracycline and yellow or brown with the
other members of the tetracycline group. The site of discoloration of the teeth depends on the age of administration of the

antibiotic, being distributed in bands around the crown. There
is some discussion as to whether the tetracycline staining is
regularly accompanied by disturbances in the formation of the
tooth tissues. If it does occur this effect must be very minor,
but it must be remembered that the disease process for which the
tetracycline had been administered might in itself cause some
disturbance in enamel or dentine formation.

A number of surveys have been carried out to investigate the
proportion of children in whom tetracycline deposition may be
found in the teeth with or without equivalent staining. The
resulting figures were surprisingly high, being over 50% in most
investigations. These statistics, however, refer to teeth in
which staining is displayed by the use of ultra-violet light to
cause fluoresence of the tetracycline. A much smaller proportion
of teeth examined at the same period showed actual discoloration.
It should be remembered that surveys of this kind, carried out in
1968 or thereabouts, are now considerably out-dated in that the
use of tetracycline in the at risk groups is now accepted as being unwise. Tetracycline staining should always be considered,
however, as a possible diagnosis within the conditions outlined.

Disturbances of Enamel and Dentine Formation
When the normal sequence of enamel matrix formation and calcification is disturbed a series of abnormalities may be produced.
These may be distinguished as hypoplasia - when the quantity of
enamel is reduced - or as hypocalcification in which the degree
of calcification is unsatisfactory. The two conditions may be
combined and various clinical conditions may be differentiated.
A parallel range of disturbances in the formation of dentine may
also occur, but these are not so well differentiated as in the
case of enamel.

The use of the term 'hypoplasia' requires some explanation,
since it is used both in the strictly scientific sense as mentioned above and also in a clinical sense to describe a generalised disturbance of enamel structure caused by some form of systemic disturbance.

This group of conditions can be conveniently divided as
follows:-

> (1) Enamel hypoplasia resulting from a local
>   or systemic disturbance during its formation.
>
> (2) Genetically determined defects of enamel
>   formation.
>
> (3) Genetically determined effects of dentine
>   formation.

Hypoplasia due to Local Infections
When an infection occurs in association with a deciduous tooth
the permanent successional tooth developing below it may undergo
a disturbance of development. In such cases the enamel is usually
distorted and pitted (Fig. 5.10). This condition is easily recog-

nized by its restriction to a single successional tooth.

Hypoplasia due to Generalized Infections and Trophic Disturbances

Widespread infections or other trophic disturbances during the tooth development period may adversely affect the laying down of enamel. Such conditions affect all the teeth developing at the time and it is often possible to time accurately the onset of the disturbance by the position of the defect on the teeth. In general the deficient enamel forms a band around the tooth corresponding to the period of disturbance (Fig. 5.11).

The band may be wide or narrow and, in some circumstances, the banding may be incomplete. It has been suggested that the enamel opacities seen in some patients may represent a minor form of this condition.

Histologically the dentine developed at the same time as the affected enamel may show slight deficiencies but this does not result in clinical abnormality.

Unless the disturbance of tooth formation is unusually severe the teeth do not seem to be unduly susceptible to attack by caries.

Prenatal syphilis may produce defects in tooth development since the spirochaete may lodge in the enamel organ and interfere directly with the formation of the enamel. In general this occurs after the differentiation of the deciduous teeth, and before the differentiation of the premolars. Thus the effects are generally confined to the anterior permanent teeth and to the first permanent molar. The typical molar form of the syphilitic tooth is the mulberry molar in which the shape of the tooth is well expressed by its name. The typical variation in the anterior teeth takes the form of a conical shape and notched incisal edge - Hutchinson's incisor (Fig. 5.12).

Hypoplasia due to Fluorosis

If the development of the teeth occurs when large amounts of fluorides are ingested mottling of the enamel may occur. The effect of fluorosis may be recognised by the presence of opaque white patches in the enamel, often arranged in a band like formation. Unlike the teeth in other forms of hypoplasia the teeth affected by fluorosis are susceptible to a brown discoloration of unknown origin which may somewhat confuse the diagnosis (Fig. 5.13). Similar idiopathic mottling may occur in teeth of patients from non-fluoride areas, but this is rare.

Amelogenesis Imperfecta

Amelogenesis imperfecta is a hereditary developmental defect of enamel. The condition may show as either a hypoplasia of the enamel or as a hypocalcification. This depends on the stage of enamel formation which is disturbed in the condition. If an early phase of enamel formation is disturbed the amount of matrix laid down is reduced but the calcification is complete. We thus have a thin and irregular layer of hard enamel. This is the

hypoplastic type.   If a later stage of enamel formation is disturbed we have a normally thick layer of poorly calcified enamel.
This is the hypocalcified type.

   In the case of hypoplasia the enamel is seen to be deficient
but hard over the whole of the dentition (Fig. 5.14).   Severe
attrition may occur early in life.   In the case of hypocalcification the whole of the enamel is soft and eroded with loss of
much enamel by attrition and exposure of the dentine (Fig. 5.15).
In both forms the deciduous and permanent dentitions may be
affected.   The dentine retains its normal structure in both
cases.

Dentinogenesis Imperfecta

   In this condition there is failure of development of the
dentine with normal enamel development.   It is a hereditary condition and, like amelogenesis imperfecta, occurs in the deciduous
and permanent dentitions.   The teeth are usually of normal morphology but grey or brown in colour (Fig. 5.16).   They show a
rather irridescent coloration which leads to the term hereditary
opalescent dentine.   The pulp chambers of affected teeth are
often reduced in size compared to the normal and may, in fact,
be obliterated.   Although the enamel is of normal structure it
readily breaks away, leaving the dentine exposed.

   Occasionally this condition occurs as part of a generalized
condition of osteogenesis imperfecta in which imperfect calcification of the bones leads to frequent fractures.   Often in such
cases there is a deficiency in the sclera of the eye leading to
a blue coloration.   This does not occur in simple cases of dentinogenesis imperfecta.

Hypoplasia associated with Generalised Disease

   Hypoplasia or hypocalcification of the enamel may occur in
patients suffering from generalised ectodermal disease (such as
epidermolysis bullosa) or from disturbances of calcium metabol-
ism such as hypoparathyroidism.   These conditions clearly represent the final result of abnormal tooth germ formation and
abnormal calcification respectively.   Many other diseases may
produce dental abnormalities of a similar type.   These changes
are, however, rare.   It is unlikely that the generalised disease
process will have gone unrecognised by the time that the tooth
abnormality has become evident in the majority of these patients
(Fig. 5.17).

   It will be evident that the diagnosis of the abnormalities of
tooth structure described above depends largely on the recognition of the clinical appearance of the teeth.   Radiography apart,
there is very little in the way of supplementary tests or investigations which will add to a carefully carried out clinical
examination of the patient - an examination which should evidently include a careful medical and family history.   In virtually all cases laboratory tests prove unproductive.

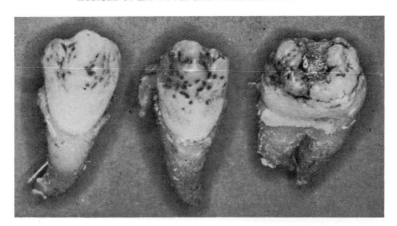

Fig. 5.10. Three teeth (not from the same patient) showing hypoplastic enamel, the result of
infection associated with a deciduous tooth.

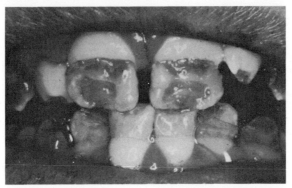

Fig. 5.11. Hypoplastic enamel resulting from a
generalised disturbance during the developmental
period. The band-like distribution is typical.

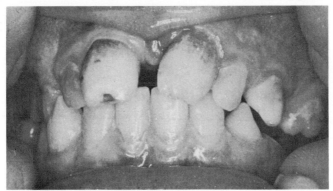

Fig. 5.12. Hutchinson's incisor of congenital
syphilis.

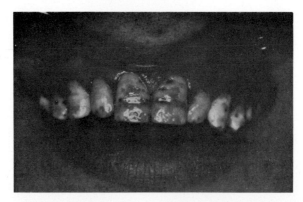

Fig. 5.13. Hypoplasia due to fluorosis. The
patient illustrated was born in a Mediterranean
island with a very high fluoride content in the
water supply.

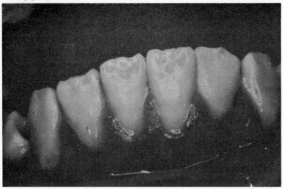

Fig. 5.14. Hypoplastic enamel. In this mild
case the enamel is evidently deficient but is
hard.

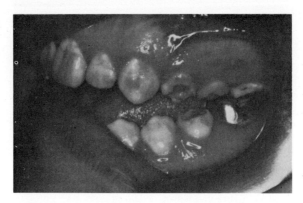

Fig. 5.15. Hypocalcified enamel. In this case
the enamel is soft and eroded.

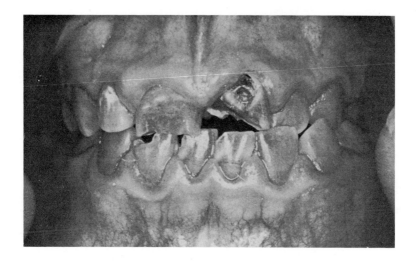

Fig. 5.16. Dentinogenesis imperfecta. Enamel
has broken away from the imperfect dentine.

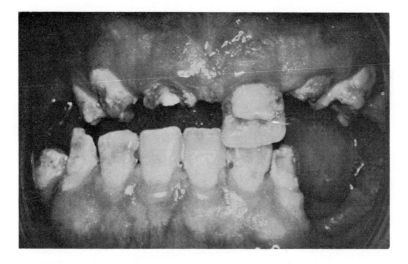

Fig. 5.17. Hypoplasia due to calcium deficiency.
In this very rare case abnormal calcium metabol-
ism has resulted in defective tooth formation.

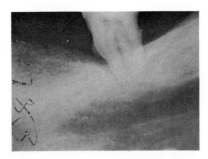

Fig. 5.18. Horizontal bone loss. The alveolar
crest bone has been lost over a wide area.

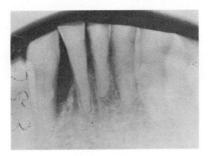

Fig. 5.19. Vertical bone loss. In this case
the bone loss is relatively localized and extends apically.

Caries
     The technique of examination of the teeth for the presence of
caries has been described in Chapter I. It must be reiterated
that an orderly and methodical plan for a visual and a probe
examination of each tooth should be adopted and adhered to as a
routine procedure, and that an accurate examination is more satis-
factorily carried out after the removal of calculus and the carrying out of prophylatic measures, followed by the drying of the
teeth. Supplemental to the clinical examination well positioned
radiographs are valuable especially in the detection of unsusp-
ected interproximal recurrent caries below fillings. Full mouth
bite wing radiographs, carefully positioned, are helpful for a
complete and accurate assessment of the patient. It should
always be remembered, however, that although the radiographs may
show cavities undetected visually or by the probe, superimposition of structures may occur and may well mask small cavities,
particularly those occurring occlusally. Radiographic examination alone cannot replace a careful clinical examination of the
patient.

     It has been shown that under standard conditions different
observers may arrive at different conclusions regarding the presence or absence of caries in the case of early occlusal lesions -
the so-called sticky fissure. This implies not a differing standard of care in examination, but a differing interpretation of
the significance of the marginal case where the carious process
is minimal. It has been also shown that the degree of sharpness
of the examining probe has a significant effect on a diagnosis in
such cases.

     The fact that the techniques available for the detection of
caries are simple must not lead to the assumption that they may
be carelessly carried out. A meticulous examination for the
presence of carious cavities is an essential preliminary to the
examination of any patient presenting with unusual or obscure
oral symptoms or complaining of facial pain of whatever distribution or degree of severity. Only after simple lesions of the
type of carious cavities have been excluded should more complex
aetiologies for pain symptoms be considered.

Pulpal Conditions and Vitality Tests
     Pain is frequently the leading symptom in pathological cond-
itions of the pulp. In the case of acute inflammation of the
pulp the pain is generally intense and may be throbbing, although
not necessarily localized within the tooth of origin. In the
case of chronic pulp conditions the pain is more likely to be
dull and to vary in its intensity over longer periods of time. In
the case of the acute conditions the response to external stimuli
of heat and cold is likely to be greater than in the case of the
chronic conditions. It is, however, not always possible to apply
these rules and there are often variations in the pain pattern
arising from similar aetiological factors. The pain of periodontitis, due to inflammatory change within the periodontal membrane,
is dissimilar from that of pulpitis in that its leading symptom
is a sensitivity of the tooth to contact, pressure or percussion.

In cases of inflammation of the pulp, however, there is frequently an associated periodontitis and it may well be that at some
stages of the process the periodontitic symptoms predominate.

Frequently pulp pathology, particularly of a chronic or degenerative type, may be associated with no pain symptoms whatever.
It must also be remembered that an attack of pulpal pain may be
terminated by death of the pulp, and by the development of a
consequent periapical lesion, the latter part of this process
being quite painless. Thus, when it is particularly important
to investigate the possibility of any dental pathology (as in
the case for instance of a rheumatic condition or a pyrexia of
unknown origin) it is essential that full mouth radiographs be
taken to include all periapical areas. Infected granulomatous
lesions may well be present without symptoms of any kind. A
greyish discoloration of the tooth is often a guide to a dead
pulp, but this is by no means a constant sign. However, discoloration of a single tooth should always be viewed with suspicion
and steps taken to ascertain the true pulpal condition.

Of the tests applicable to determine the condition of a pulp
the most widely applied is the electric pulp tester. In its
most usual form the electric pulp tester consists of a device
whereby an alternating current is passed through the tooth, the
applied voltage being varied. The voltage level to which the
pulp responds by producing pain symptoms is used as a measure of
the degree of vitality of the pulp.

The voltage of the alternating current may be either quite
low (12-24 volts) or may be very much higher (up to 2,000 volts).
The basic frequency used is of the order of up to 200 cycles/
second.

In a second form of electric pulp tester the stimulus applied
is a variable direct current, the painful response of the tooth
as the current is increased being used as the measure of vitality.

When using one of these instruments the tooth in question,
adjacent teeth and soft tissues should be dry and care taken to
ensure good contact of the electrode on to sound tooth substance.
The results obtained from comparative use of these pulp testers
under different conditions on different teeth often appear to be
widely divergent. However, with a standardized technique and
careful handling, the electric pulp tester may be used to give a
good comparative picture of the pulp vitality and reaction,
although it is difficult to say from any single pulp test of a
tooth what is the precise condition of the pulp. Whatever form
the pulp test may take it should always be the practice to similarly test adjacent teeth and the equivalent tooth in the opposite quadrant of the mouth in order to gain some idea of the reaction of the presumably normal teeth. In general a completely
non-reactive tooth implies pulp death. A normal reading, i.e.
one comparable with other similar teeth, does not necessarily
imply a normal pulp, as chronically inflamed or otherwise

abnormal pulps may well give a normal reading. It is probably
wisest to accept all evidence from the simple electric pulp
testers at present commercially available as being to some degree
fallible.

     The application of heat or cold to a tooth may give a good
indication of pulp death in the case of non-reaction. Heat may
be applied by a heated burnisher or a heated fragment of gutta
percha. Great care must be taken in the application of hot
testing instruments that an involuntary movement of the patient
does not result in a burn on the lip or cheek. Reaction to cold
is best measured by the application of ethyl chloride via a well-
soaked cotton wool pledgelet. As in the case of the electric
pulp test, some attempt must be made to establish a normal reaction by similarly testing adjacent teeth and teeth in the opposite
quadrant. Although testing by heat or cold is a limited technique, it is quite reliable within its limitations, i.e. the recognition of non-vital pulps. No vitality test gives any more reliable information.

     In some instances a widely exposed and hence inflamed pulp
reacts in a hyperplastic manner and expands by the production of
granulation tissue which protrudes through the carious cavity.
This occurs only in teeth where large apical foramina allow of a
free blood supply. This is in effect restricted to deciduous
molars, first permanent molars and very occasionally permanent
incisors. The polyp, lying in the carious cavity, often resembles
an inflamed and hyperplastic gingival papilla. It may be at once
distinguished, however, by gentle pricking with a probe. The
polyp being virtually without sensory nerve supply, will give the
patient no pricking sensation at all. This is a useful test if
the field is slightly obscured by haemorrhage from the rather
fragile inflamed tissues.

Periapical Granuloma
     Following necrosis and infection of a pulp, toxic material and
organisms may pass through the apical foramen. If the resistance
of the tissues is high and the virulence of the infection low,
the tissue reaction may result in the formation of a granuloma.
This, a spherical mass of granulation tissue surrounding the apex,
is clinically a relatively quiescent lesion and in itself produces no pain symptoms unless secondary infection should occur.
Thus the granuloma may be associated with a tooth which is normal
in appearance. Other non-vital teeth with granulomatous lesions
may be abnormally dark in colour and may be slightly tender to
percussion. In general, however, the diagnostic weapon to detect
the presence of a periapical granuloma is the radiograph. The
typical appearance is of a discrete osteolytic lesion, apparently
spherical in shape, and not delineated by a radio-opaque margin.
This radiographic appearance is relatively constant, but there is
the possibility of confusion with anatomical structures such as
the mental foramen, the incisive foramen, or even a particularly
large bone trabecula (Fig. 1.1, Chapter I). If doubt arises, then
a second radiograph is taken from a different angle. A superimposed anatomical structure will appear to move in respect to

the apex, whilst a periapical lesion continues to give its typical appearance.

Chronic Periapical Abscess

Should the central area of a granuloma break down as a result
of continuing low-grade infection, then a chronic abscess is
formed with the production of pus. In such a case the process
may be quite painless although there may be some sensitivity of
the tooth to percussion and also tenderness of the alveolus to
pressure over the apex. Frequently such lesions show periodic
exacerbations in which, for a short time, dull pain is felt and
the sensitivity to percussion is increased.

A common consequence of a chronic abscess is the formation of
a sinus with discharge of pus to an external surface. In most
cases this discharge of pus occurs through the cortical bone to
the nearest available surface - often this is the buccal alveolar
surface, although this depends on the precise local anatomy. A
chronic abscess on the palatal root of a maxillary molar, for
instance, might be expected to discharge palatally. Sinus formation is occasionally periodic in nature and closure of the sinus
may be associated with an exacerbation of pain which is again
reduced with re-opening of the sinus.

Occasionally the pus may track for some distance before penetrating the surface. The most frequently seen example of this
is in the case of an abscess on a maxillary lateral incisor from
which pus may track posteriorly to form a sinus orifice in the
palate nearby the first permanent molar. If the anatomical factors are such as to allow it, the pus may discharge extraorally.
The most common site for this is the mandibular incisor region,
where an apical abscess may form an external sinus opening on the
chin. Such an externally opening sinus may be associated with
buried roots in an otherwise edentulous mouth and a chronic sinus
of this kind should always be investigated radiographically for
the presence of retained roots.

A sinus orifice, particularly when newly opened, may present a
rolled and hyperplastic appearance of either mucous membrane or
skin which may easily be mistaken for a neoplastic growth. A
well-established sinus orifice on the mucosa may bear a considerable resemblance to an aphthous ulcer. Diagnosis in both cases
is by the presence of actively discharging pus through a patent
sinus, and the radiographic evidence of the underlying periapical
lesion.

Acute Periapical Abscess

An acute periapical infection most often results from invasion
of the tissues by organisms introduced via a non-vital pulp. This
invasion of the periapical regions may be consequent either on a
long-standing chronic condition or may arise following acute
trauma of sufficient intensity to cause pulp death. The early
symptoms of such an acute lesion depend on inflammatory changes
in the periodontal membrane which occur, at this stage, without
any recognizable radiographic change in the periapical bone. If

the resistance of the tissues is insufficient to overcome the
virulence of the invading organism then the process may advance
to pus formation, to bone resorption and the consequent eventual
radiographic recognition of bone loss.

The leading symptom is usually severe pain over the area of
the infection. The pain is frequently described as throbbing in
nature and is often associated with great sensitivity of the
tooth to percussion. The tooth may be lifted appreciably from
its socket by the hyperaemia of the periodontal membrane and
thereby become mobile. The overlying tissues are frequently red
and swollen. At this stage in the inflammatory process the recognition of the condition is rarely difficult in view of the
sensitivity of the tooth concerned. Extraction of the tooth at
this stage may show an apical mass of tissue which is either a
secondary infected granulomatous lesion or a primitive abscess
sac formed in an attempt to restrict further spread of the infection.

Acute Alveolar Abscess
Following acute inflammation of the periapical tissues, unless
resolution occurs, spread of the infection takes place to the
surrounding alveolar tissues and an acute alveolar abscess is
formed. In the early stages the marrow spaces of the alveolar
bone are filled by pus under pressure and pain is intense and
throbbing. Adjacent teeth may also become involved and become
highly sensitive to percussion.

The next stage is perforation of the alveolar bone by the pus.
Often this results in an immediate, if temporary, reduction of
the pain symptoms. The site of perforation of the bone depends
on the precise local anatomy of the area. In particular, the
relationship of the apex of the tooth to nearby muscle attach-
ments and fascial planes determines the extent of the area of
subsequent tissue involvement as the spread of pus is bounded to
a considerable extent by these structures.

The significant structure in the posterior maxilla is the buccinator muscle, attached to the lateral aspect of the maxilla
along a line at approximately the level of the molar apices. If
pus perforates above this line it may spread upwards towards the
infratemporal fossa. Pus perforating below this line will appear
in the buccal sulcus. The equivalent tissue barrier in the anterior part of the maxilla is provided by the levator labii and
associated muscles. Generally pus tracking from an anterior
tooth will perforate below the insertions of these muscles but
very occasionally perforates above them where it is diverted into
the infra-orbital area.

The significant structure in the mandible is the mylohyoid
muscle separating the sublingual and submandibular spaces. Lingual perforation of pus from the apices of second and third molars
normally occurs below the mylohyoid line and leads to a submandibular infection. Anteriorly to this the apices of the teeth lie
above the oblique mylohyoid line and lingual perforation results

in sublingual infection.

The buccinator muscle may also occasionally prove a barrier
to pus produced in the mandibular third molar area. Since the
attachment of the muscle is lost in the area of the first molar,
pus produced posteriorly may track forward below the attachment
and appear in the buccal sulcus opposite the first molar. The
situation may then appear to be of an abscess pointing in close
relationship to a quite normal tooth. In this case diagnosis
may be confirmed by the sensitivity of the infected tooth to
percussion and by radiographic evidence if the acute infection is
consequent on an exacerbation of a chronic state.

Following perforation of the cortical bone pus may be for a
short time confined beneath the periosteum as a subperiosteal
abscess. In this case the surrounding soft tissues are extremely
tender with some localized oedema, but without generalized swelling. Usually, however, perforation of the periosteal layer rapidly occurs and pus is liberated into the overlying tissue space.
Following the liberation of the pus into the tissues, the first
reaction is usually one of cellulitis - a diffuse inflammatory
reaction with all the signs and symptoms of acute infection but
without localization or the formation of significant quantities
of pus. Thus it is that at this stage of an acute infection surgical intervention produces little in the way of drainage since
the inflammatory process is diffused throughout the tissues.
However, depending on the type of organism, the vigour of the
bodily defence mechanisms and the extent of treatment applied,
the next stage in the progress of the inflammatory process consists of a localization of the inflammatory products with the
formation of pus.

It is normally only at this stage that pus may be obtained by
incision or aspiration. It follows that identification of the
organism responsible for the infection is almost impossible until
this stage is reached. Thus, unfortunately, it is necessary to
proceed with treatment along arbitrary lines whilst the tissues
are in the state of cellulitis. If the infection is due to a
non-pyogenic organism such as a haemolytic streptococcus, then
material can rarely be obtained for bacteriological examination.

Non-odontogenic Infections
It must be remembered that infections of a non-odontogenic
origin occurring about the face may simulate dental infections.
A boil in the early stage of cellulitis may resemble an acute
alveolar abscess, but the ready pointing and its lack of association with a periostitic tooth should give a clue as to its non-
odontogenic origin. Swellings of the soft tissues of the face
and neck are discussed more fully in Chapter IX.

Lesions of the Periodontal Tissues

There is no generally accepted system of nomenclature of periodontal disease and it is necessary to define certain terms before discussion of the diagnosis of the clinical entities.

Gingivitis is inflammation of the gingival tissues without involvement of the periodontal tissues of attachment. The exact site of this inflammatory process may be indicated by the terms marginal or papillary. A variation in the balance of the inflammatory mechanism producing exuberant fibrous tissue is termed hyperplastic gingivitis.

Periodontitis represents an extension of the inflammatory process to the periodontal ligament and the supporting bone.

A pocket is the result of apical migration of the epithelium of attachment of a tooth, leading to abnormal deepening of the gingival sulcus. A false pocket is produced by hyperplastic change in the gingivae which thereby grows and produces a pocket without apical migration of the epithelium of attachment.

Horizontal bone loss implies resorption of alveolar crest bone, often fairly uniformly over a wide area (Fig. 5.18).

Vertical bone loss implies bone resorption occurring in an apical direction along the root of a tooth or teeth and appears in effect as an extension of a deep pocket into the bone. Such a pocket is an intrabony pocket (Fig. 5.19).

Among the factors to be considered in the diagnosis of periodontal conditions are the following:-

(i)   Age and Sex of the Patient.
        These are of considerable significance in that several periodontal lesions, although not perhaps under direct hormonal control, are certainly affected by changes in hormonal balance. Puberty in both sexes, pregnancy and the female menopause are periods of particular significance.

(ii)   The Presence of Plaque.
        This is perhaps one of the most important factors in the aetiology of periodontal disease. Its presence may be demonstrated by the use of dyes in disclosing solutions or tablets - erythrosin is the most commonly used of these. A number of rather arbitrary indices have been devised for the recording, not only of plaque, but also of calculus and of the damage caused by periodontal disease. These are of use in dental health research projects and in the assessment of treatment rather than in diagnosis.

(iii)   The Presence of Calculus.
        This is of great aetiological importance in periodontal disease but is by no means present in all conditions. Supragingival calculus is readily visible but subgingival deposits must be carefully sought for with the aid of a Briault probe which readily differentiates the rough texture of the calculus. Subgingival calculus may be often visualized by blowing the

gingival sulcus away from the tooth surface with
the compressed air syringe.

(iv)   The Presence of Pockets.
        Some degree of pocketing is normal and the depth of
        pockets may be measured by the use of a graduated
        flat seeker. In what is regarded as a normal
        mouth, a pocket depth of up to 2 mm is to be expec-
        ted, this representing the physiological depth of
        the gingival crevice together with the minor degree
        of true pocket formation which is almost universal.

(v)   The Colour and Texture of the Gingivae.
        The colour of normal gingival tissue is pink and
        the texture firm and resilient to pressure. Inflam-
        matory changes are often shown by a hyperaemia
        producing a smooth red appearance of the gingivae
        together with oedema which reduces the resilient
        texture and allows of pitting on pressure.

(vi)   Fragility of the Gingivae.
        Contact and gentle pressure on a normal gingival
        margin produces no ill effect. In disease, however,
        haemorrhage is often freely produced by quite light
        pressure. In conditions in which the epithelial
        layer tends to become detached from the underlying
        corium gentle wiping movements with gauze or cotton
        wool may cause the epithelium to slip off leaving a
        rather raw area. This is Nikolsky's sign.

(vii)   The Presence of Ulceration or Pus.
        Pus within a pocket may be demonstrated by gentle
        pressure on the tissues. Lesser quantities are
        best demonstrated on a probe or seeker introduced
        into the pocket.

(viii) Bone Loss as Measured Radiographically.
        Periapical radiographs are a considerable help in
        the assessment of bone destruction. There may,
        however, be difficulties in interpretation due to
        superimposition of, say a high lingual bone crest
        over a resorbed buccal bone area. In such a case
        the bone loss may be undetected. Introduction of a
        radiopaque foreign body to the depths of a bony
        pocket - a gutta percha or silver point, a wire or
        a probe end - will demonstrate the true degree of
        bone loss.

(ix)   Tooth Mobility.
        Testing for mobility has been discussed in Chapter
        I.

(x)   Percussion.
        When struck gently by an instrument (most commonly
        with a reversed mirror handle) a tooth emits a per-
        cussion sound dependent on the degree of alveolar

support - the less the support, the higher the
note. At the same time a finger placed against
the tooth can register minor degrees of movement.
Evidently the tooth or teeth in question should be
percussed together with others for comparative
purposes.

(xi)   Halitosis.
Some periodontal conditions produce a quite characteristic halitosis. In others secondary infection, the gathering of food debris in pockets and
lack of oral hygiene may result in a strong, but
not specific, mouth odour.

(xii)   Occlusal disharmony.
Abnormalities in occlusion, localized malposition-
ing of teeth and occlusal irregularity caused by
restorations must be noted. Study models are
often a help in assessing these factors. Full
occlusal analysis may be carried out using an
anatomical articulator to mount the models, although this is not a usual requirement. Labial
incompetence leading to mouthbreathing should be
noted.

(xiii) Systematic disease.
The patient should be questioned as to the possibility of any previously diagnosed diseases.

(xiv)   Drugs.
Any drugs regularly taken by the patient should be
identified. Oral contraceptives may be particularly significant.

(xv)   Restorations.
The restorations present in filled or crowned
teeth should be examined in respect of satisfactory occlusion and interproximal contour. Doubtful
gingival ledges may be shown up radiographically.

   Although there is a wide spectrum of possible manifestations
of chronic periodontal disease there are certain well recognized
clinical entities into which the vast majority of conditions fall.
The diagnostic criteria associated with these conditions include
reference to all the previously mentioned considerations.

Chronic Inflammatory Conditions

(i)   Chronic Gingivitis.
Chronic gingivitis - usually marginal - is widely
present amongst adults of both sexes. Examination
shows the presence of plaque and of calculus sub-
gingivally and often supragingivally. Pocketing
is present up to 3 mm in depth. The gingival
margins are red, spongy and with a tendency to
bleed. Ulceration and pus are absent and generally

speaking the condition is quite painless. There
is no bone loss and no increased mobility of the
teeth since the periodontal tissues of attachment
are not affected but some patients may complain of
gingival recession and there may be gingival
detachment. There is no specific halitosis although the patient may complain of a bad taste or
bad breath. Irregularity of arch form and poorly
contoured restorations may be of great significance in causing local inflammation.

(ii)   Chronic Hyperplastic Gingivitis.
In this condition - fundamentally similar to
chronic marginal gingivitis - the proliferative
element of the inflammatory process dominates and
fibrous hyperplasia of the gingivae occurs. It
may occur at any age and in either sex, but there
is an increased tendency to this condition at
puberty. Plaque and subgingival calculus are
present. Both true pocketing and false pocketing
due to overgrowth of the gingivae is present.
Because of the increased fibrous component in the
tissues the gingivae are usually pale and firm
although secondary infection within the deep pockets may cause redness and fragility of the tissues. Similarly ulceration and pus occurs in the
pockets after secondary infection. The condition
is painless unless secondary infection occurs and
there is no bone loss or tooth mobility. Non-
specific halitosis due to food stagnation may
occur. Occlusal malrelationships and lip incompetence leading to mouthbreathing potentiate the
condition. The condition occurs in a marked form
in approximately 50 per cent of patients taking
the drug epanutin (phenytoin sodium, dilantin).
In this case the hyperplastic reaction is papillary rather than marginal. The degree to which
epanutin induced gingivitis is due to the drug
alone is uncertain since extremely strict attention to oral hygiene may reduce the severity of the
condition greatly. It would seem that the condition represents an acceleration of the normal
pathology of chronic gingivitis. Histologically
there are some differences in that the degree of
fibrous hyperplasia and also of epithelial hyperplasia in the affected areas is greater than in
the usual hyperplastic gingivitis.

     During pregnancy a previously existing chronic
gingivitis may be exacerbated and somewhat modified under the influence of hormonal changes.
There may be only minimal amounts of calculus
present. Pockets are formed which are largely
false since the characteristic of the condition is
a hyperplastic reaction of the gingivae and particularly of the papillae. The reaction is much

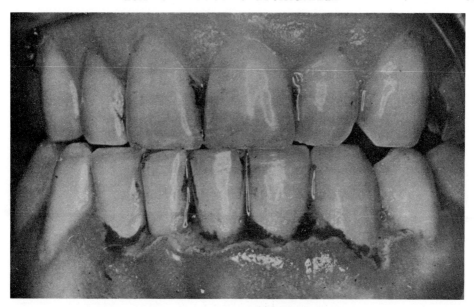

Fig. 5.20. Early acute ulcerative gingivitis.
Ulceration of the gingival papillae and lateral
extension is evident.

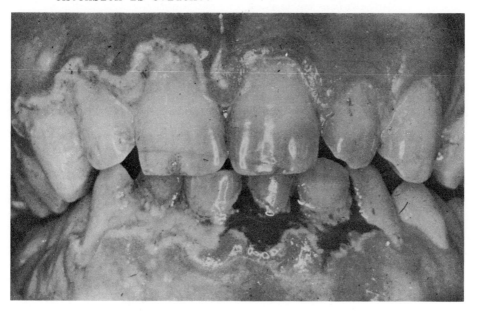

Fig. 5.21. In this later case ulceration is
more advanced and papillary necrosis is evident.

less fibrous than in other hyperplastic conditions
and the tissue contains many rather primitive capillaries and even blood spaces. The papillae appear
purple-red and irregular with a spongy texture and
tend to bleed with very light trauma. Pus is present
only if secondary infection occurs and there is no
pain. There is no bone loss or mobility of the teeth.
Halitosis is present only as a secondary feature due
to food stagnation.

An occasional feature is the growth of one single
papilla to form a mass of granulation tissue known as
a pregnancy tumour or pregnancy epulis. Such a lesion
may be the only gingival manifestation of the pregnancy. The lesion may grow quite large, up to 2 cm.
diameter. Diagnosis is by the history and by confirmatory excision biopsy. This latter procedure is
fraught with some difficulty as the lesion may be
excessively haemorrhagic and, since the mass is likely
to regress considerably, if not completely after pregnancy, there is something to be said for leaving the
lesion temporarily in place. The purple colour, rapid
growth, site and timing of the occurrence of the lesion is sufficient for a strong presumptive diagnosis.
However, if there is the slightest doubt as to the
nature of the growth then biopsy excision is indicated
and the pregnancy itself must be counted as no contra-
indication to this.

A similar state may occur at puberty when an
upsurge in hormonal activity, not unlike that during
pregnancy, may accentuate a previous chronic gingivitis. This condition resolves after puberty. Women
on oral contraceptives may show a similar gingivitis.

(iii) Chronic Periodontitis
This condition may be subdivided into two forms
(simplex and complex) which are essentially the same,
but which differ in the degree of tissue involvement.

Simplex periodontal disease (periodontitis simplex)
is an inflammatory process in which the changes which
affect the gingivae in chronic gingivitis are extended
to include the periodontal membrane and supporting
alveolar bone. Subgingival calculus is present extending deep into the pockets. The pockets are intrabony
and more than 3 mm deep - often much more. The colour,
texture and fragility of the gingivae are as in chronic
gingivitis, but with the redness, spongy texture and
fragility somewhat increased - pus is generally present in the pockets. Bone loss of the horizontal type
may be seen on radiographic examination and loss of
support leads to tooth mobility. A non-specific
halitosis results from the infected pockets.

Complex periodontal disease (periodontitis complex)

represents an extension of the processes of chronic
periodontitis with deep pocketing and vertical bone
loss.   It tends to be rapidly progressive, leading to
early tooth mobility.

Epulides. An epulis is, simply, a swelling on the gingival
margin. The term is used to describe a range of hyperplastic
inflammatory lesions arising from the periodontium and presenting
as discrete single swellings. They represent in structure a
pathological extension of the normal metabolic functions of the
periodontal tissues. They occur over a very wide age range, from
very young to very old, and there is no sex differentiation.

The swelling arises interdentally from the periodontal membrane. There is, at an early stage, some resorption of crest
bone which may become much greater with increased growth and
especially in the presence of secondary infection. There are
three well-defined types. A fibrous epulis is the result of
exuberant fibrous tissue formation. It is pink in colour and
firm in texture, with no tendency to bleed. A giant cell epulis
(myeloid epulis) contains many foreign body giant cells distributed in a connective tissue stroma with many capillaries. It is
purple in colour, rather fragile and with a tendency to bleed.
The third type of commonly seen epulis is the pyogenic granuloma.
This presents as an irregular growth of exuberant, rather
immature, granulation tissue with many capillaries and even blood
spaces. It is red in colour, fragile and bleeds easily. The
pregnancy epulis is a form of this lesion. These lesions show
different facets of the same process but, although there may be
specimens which are somewhat transitional in type, the classification is well marked and usually quite distinct.

Diagnosis is by excision biopsy. Examination of the tissue of
an excised epulis is quite essential since, very rarely, the
appearance of an epulis is presented by a secondary neoplasm.   In
general, further investigations of the patients are not called
for but an exception to this is the case of the giant cell
epulis.   In a few patients such a lesion may occur as a response
to hyperparathyroidism (in itself, usually caused by a neoplasm
of the parathyroids).   This being so, it is necessary to screen
such patients to ensure a normal serum calcium, phosphorus and
alkaline phosphatase (Chapters II and VII).   If these are abnormal then suspicions of parathyroid abnormality should be aroused.

Acute Inflammatory Conditions
    Unlike the position in chronic gingival inflammations where
the significance of bacterial or viral activity is unknown,
there are specific acute gingival conditions associated with the
presence of various types of organism. Localized acute periodontitis, however, is not generally associated with any specific
organism or group of organisms and may, indeed, be a non-infected
process.

    Acute ulcerative gingivitis (acute necrotizing gingivitis).
The aetiology of this condition is far from clear in that, although there is invariably a great overgrowth of the Vincent's
organisms Borrelia vincenti and Fusiformis fusiformis, there is
no clear evidence that these are the primary infecting agents.
Both unspecified viruses and bacterioiedes melaninogenicus have
been implicated as the primary agent, but without much evidence.
However, from a diagnostic point of view it is safe to say that
an attack of acute ulcerative gingivitis is characterized by the
presence of the Vincent's organisms in very large numbers. It
should be pointed out that these organisms, in much smaller numbers, are commensal inhabitants of many normal mouths.

    An attack of ulcerative gingivitis is not confined to any age
group or sex, but tends to occur in the young adult age group.
There is not necessarily a previous high degree of calculus formation or of pocketing, although poor oral hygiene is frequently a
potentiating factor in the disease. The gingivae are, in a fully
developed case, red, spongy, extremely tender and bleeding. There
is ulceration of the gingival papilla. This is of a rather rapid
necrotic type in which the papilla may be eroded almost completely away. The ulceration of the papillae may extend laterally to
include virtually the whole gingival margin (Figs. 5.20, 5.21).
The saucer-shaped ulcers of the papillae are highly diagnostic.
There is a quite characteristic halitosis in this condition. Direct smears of the ulcerated areas show the Vincent's organisms on
gram staining. Culture of the organisms is difficult and is not
attempted as a routine diagnostic procedure.

    The initial point of infection may be associated with stagnat-
ion areas resulting from overcrowding or, particularly a pericor-
onitic area around a partially erupted tooth. There is often
malaise, a rise in temperature of a few degrees, and submandibular lymphadentitis occurring with or after the commencement of the
oral symptoms.

    The ulceration may in severe cases be transmitted by contact
to the oral mucous membrane. In extremely severe and rare cases
the infection and ulceration may include a considerable area of
the oral and oro-pharangeal mucosa - the condition known as Vincent's angina.

    In tropical conditions and in patients with a poor standard of
nutrition the infective process may erode completely through the
buccal tissues. This fulminating form of Vincent's infection is
known as Cancrum oris.

Recurrence of acute ulcerative gingivitis is not unusual and is most often associated with continuing poor oral hygiene. It may, however, be associated with systemic disease - especially the blood dyscrasias - and the patient whose symptoms fail to respond to treatment or in whom there are unexplained recurrences should be investigated by blood examination.

Acute herpetic gingivitis and acute streptococcal gingivitis are discussed in Chapter VI.

Acute periodontitis. Acute periodontitis is a condition normally confined to one or a very few teeth. The symptoms are due to inflammatory changes in the periodontal membrane leading to raising of the tooth from its normal position. Aetiological factors include acute trauma to the tooth, apical extension of the inflammatory process from an acutely inflamed pulp, spread of toxic material or organisms from a non-vital pulp, diffusion of chemicals used in endodontic procedures, foreign bodies introduced into the periodontal tissues or interdental space and occlusal traumatism from high fillings. Symptoms include premature contact, tenderness to percussion and mobility. In the early stages tenderness may be relieved by gentle pressure on the tooth, although this stage is soon replaced by one of great sensitivity. If the aetiological factor is the extension of the inflammatory reaction from an acutely inflamed pulp then the tooth will display the thermal sensitivity and pulp testing reactions of acute pulpitis. If occlusal traumatism following conservative treatment is the cause, then a highly polished facet may be seen on the occlusal surface of the filling.

Diagnosis is from these symptoms, with the confirmation of an aetiological factor which may often be determined. Radiographs may show no change or may show a little widening of the normal thickness of the periodontal membrane.

Acute periodontal abscess. A periodontal abscess is an abscess of the periodontal tissues only, not affecting the pulp or periapical tissues, and having the gingival sulcus as the point of entry of the organisms responsible. It is frequently the result of an acute exacerbation of a chronic periodontal condition.

Since local tissue reaction, pain, tenderness to percussion, lymphadenitis and malaise may closely simulate a periapical abscess it is important to make a careful differentiation between the two. In the case of the periodontal abscess the tooth will respond to vitality testing unless some other factor is involved. Radiographs show no periapical changes, although alveolar bone loss and intrabony pocketing may be seen. Caries or fillings may be completely absent from the tooth.

The differential diagnosis depends on recognition of the fact that the periapical abscess is essentially a lesion of a non-vital tooth, whereas a periodontal abscess is not.

Pericoronitis. Pericoronitis is a periodontal abscess occurring in the tissues overlying a partially erupted tooth -

especially a third molar. The tissues surrounding and overlying
the tooth appear red, swollen and extremely tender and there is
often pus lying within the gingival trough distal to an affected
third molar. An operculum lying partly over the occlusal surface
of the tooth is often seen, red, oedematous and intensely painful
to touch. The infection frequently extends to the surrounding
soft tissues and there is pain, oedema, submandibular lymphadenitis, pyrexia, malaise and trismus.

The infecting organism is, in general, non-specific but may in
some cases have all the characteristics of a Vincent's infection.
In this case the pericoronitis may act as the initiating focus
for the spread of a typical acute ulcerative gingivitis.

Desquamative gingivitis
This is a term used to describe the occurrence of an erosive
or bullous condition predominantly affecting the gingiva. The
histology is of lichen planus or occasionally of pemphigoid -
conditions discussed more fully in the next chapter. In the past
it was thought that desquamative gingivitis might exist as an
entity distinct from these two conditions and there has been much
confusion. This confusion has been increased by the use of the
term 'gingivosis' as synonymous with 'desquamative gingivitis'
although it was originally used in a quite different context -
that of degenerative periodontal loss associated with malnutrit-
ion. The diagnosis may be simply confirmed by biopsy examination
but, not infrequently, biopsy of the affected gingival tissue may
lead to unacceptable loss of contour. In these circumstances it
is not unreasonable to rely on clinical factors for diagnosis.

The gingivae appear red and shiny and there are erosions on
the slightly swollen interdental papillae. Lesions of lichen
planus may be noticed on other areas of the oral mucosa, although
not invariably so. If so, they may present a more suitable site
for biopsy than the gingivae. The periodontal ligament is not
directly involved and any bone loss is due to secondary disease
consequent on the difficulty in maintaining an adequate oral
hygiene. Thus, there are no characteristic radiographic features.

Periodontosis. Periodontosis is a term used to describe a
degenerative change in the periodontal tissues leading to marked
bone loss and tooth mobility. There is continuing controversy as
to whether it, in fact, exists; some authorities considering it
to be a special case of periodontitis and not essentially degenerative in nature. Whatever the initial aetiology the clinical
diagnosis is made on the following criteria.

The patients are described as being under the age of 30, with
a preponderance of females. The dominant symptom is tooth mobility which is seen on radiographic examination to be due to excessive thickening of the periodontal ligament. A characteristic
feature is migration of the teeth in a manner not associated with
occlusal stress. The gingivae appear substantially normal in the
early stages; there is no ulceration or pus present and no pain.
In later stages inflammatory changes are superimposed and there

is increasing gingival inflammation and pocketing. At this stage
the findings resemble those of advanced periodontitis with marked
bone loss. No systemic disturbance has been described as being
associated with this condition.

Fibromatosis (gingival hyperplasia). This is a non-inflammat-
ory hyperplastic condition in which the fibrous tissue of the
gingival corium becomes enormously increased in volume. The
condition would appear to be genetically determined.

The overgrowth of tissue usually begins at an early age -
three to four years - although it may be present from the eruption
of the deciduous dentition or may be delayed in appearance until
puberty. Secondary infection is common, with the presence of
calculus and, in view of the nature of the condition, deep false
pockets. The gingivae are pale pink in colour and firm in texture. Pus is present only with secondary infection in a pocket.
There is no pain except for secondary infection. Similarly, bone
loss and tooth mobility do not form part of the original condition, but in view of the great depth of the false pockets with the
possibility of stagnation and infection, vertical bone loss may
occur. The occlusal pattern may well be profoundly influenced by
the masses of fibrous tissue which form an obstruction to the normal pattern of eruption. No systemic factors have been shown to
be associated with this condition.

Periodontal traumatism. Periodontal traumatism is the name
given to a condition brought about by abnormal and pathological
changes taking place in the periodontal tissues as a result of
occlusal stresses of abnormal intensity. These stresses are
brought about by a traumatic occlusion which may affect one or
several teeth.

Calculus is not a feature of this condition, nor are interproximal pockets. Two features of the gingival morphology in this
condition are Stillman's clefts and McCall's festoons. Stillman's
clefts are areas of severe gingival recession associated with the
labial surface of lower anterior teeth. McCall's festoons are
thick gingival rolls also placed labially on lower anterior
teeth. These occur when the direction of the trauma is directed
linguo-labially on the lower anterior teeth. The colour and texture of the gingival margins is, in general, not greatly changed.
There is no pus and no pain symptoms. Bone loss is horizontal in
nature as distinct from the vertical bone loss in periodontosis
and is maximal in the alveolar process away from the direction of
the applied stress. Mobility of the teeth due to loss of attachment occurs as does migration of the teeth. This migration of
the teeth occurs along lines determined by the occlusal stress
and not in a random manner as in periodontosis. Occlusal analysis demonstrates the incidence of the traumatic forces.

Chapter VI

Lesions of the Oral Mucosa

Lesions of the oral mucosa in general can be divided into two broad groups. In the first of these groups the lesions result from some local abnormality and there are no other systemic manifestations. In the second group, however, the oral lesion may simply represent a localised manifestation of some generalised disease process affecting the skin, other mucous membrane or apparently unrelated structures. Although this division is theoretically a simple one to make it is often difficult on clinical examination to decide whether a mucosal abnormality is, in fact, an entirely localised one. Many of the problems in the diagnosis of these lesions stem from the necessity to make sure that a more widespread condition is not involved. For this reason the medical history takes on a particular importance when dealing with patients with such lesions.

As has been pointed out in Chapter I, the patient may have great difficulty in realising the significance of medical details apparently unrelated to an abnormality occurring within the mouth and it is often necessary to ask direct questions. When doing so certain special relationships must be borne in mind - for instance, that between the skin and the mucous membrane. Although the oral mucous membrane is histologically similar to other lining mucosae it behaves in some respects as a modified form of skin and a considerable number of skin diseases show lesions in the mouth. It is not unusual for the earliest lesions of such conditions to appear in the mouth and thus present an opportunity for diagnosis. The oral mucous membrane also bears considerable similarities, both histological and immunological, to the genital and opthalmic mucosae. It is consequentially not uncommon for similar lesions to affect more than one of these structures.

The relationship of the oral mucosa to the lower gastro-intestinal tract mucosae is less direct. This is presumably dependent on the differing structure and functions of the lining membrane of the mouth compared to the lower gut mucosa with their secretory and absorptive functions. There are a few conditions, however, in which there appears to be a direct relationship between lower gut lesions and those in the mouth. An example of this is the occurrence of oral ulceration in patients with ulcerative colitis - such ulceration may be very severe and associated with similar lesions of the skin. In these circumstances it is presumed that a similar mechanism affects both mucosae and the skin. In other circumstances the relationship between oral and lower gut abnormality may be indirect and the result of malabsorption problems. Patients with an association of this type include those with stomatitis arising from anaemias and

nutritional defects of various kinds. A further group of oral
lesions also bears an indirect relationship with lower gut
abnormality via a common association with certain HLA loci - it
would seem likely that the association between recurrent oral
ulceration and coeliac disease may be of this type.

Not only lower gastro-intestinal disorders but many others may
be associated with lesions in the mouth and it is evident that
anyone dealing with these conditions must have a wide general
knowledge of medical and surgical pathology extending well beyond
the limits of the mouth itself.

It is quite impossible to suggest a complete scheme of
screening procedures suitable for every possible oral mucosal
lesion. The steps to be taken depend on the clinical examination
- it would evidently be completely uneconomic to carry out a full
range of screening tests and procedures in every case. In the
majority of cases the most important single diagnostic procedure
is the taking of a biopsy, and in most instances this is sufficient to confirm a diagnosis in cases of doubt.

Certain important groups of oral lesions are considered below
and diagnostic techniques appropriate to these groups are
outlined.

Recurrent Oral Ulceration (R.O.U.)

Although many lesions of the oral mucosa are both recurrent
and ulcerative the term 'recurrent oral ulceration' is used to
describe a well defined group of conditions which are well known
and common, some twenty to twenty five per cent of the population being affected by them at some time. The initial diagnosis
is almost entirely clinical and relies heavily on the history as
given by the patient. Although there is a spectrum of presentations and although the groups are not absolutely clear cut, the
great majority of the patients with R.O.U. can be placed into
one of three classifications.

Minor aphthous ulceration. In this, the commonest variant,
the usual pattern is from one to six ulcers appearing at a time.
The onset of minor aphthous ulceration (as well as other forms of
R.O.U.) may be at any age - small children may be affected and
there is no proved increase in incidence at adolescence. The
size is variable, usually of the order of 2 to 5 millimetres in
diameter, although some may be occasionally larger. The duration
is of the order of ten days after which the ulcers heal without
scarring. There is then a variable free period which may range
from a matter of days to many months before a further attack.
Stress may be implicated in precipitating the attacks in some,
but not all, patients. These ulcers virtually never affect the
palatal mucosa or the throat.

Major aphthous ulceration. In this form there is a variable
number of ulcers which are predominantly larger than those of
the minor variety. The characteristic feature is, however, the

length of time for which they may last - months in some instances
- and the tissue destruction and scarring which may sometimes be
caused. There is usually no recognisable cyclic pattern. Any
site in the mouth and oro pharynx may be affected.

   Herpetiform ulcers. In this variant a large number of very
small but painful ulcers appear in batches. The duration is
variable - usually of the order of one to two weeks. The most
common site is at the floor of the mouth and the lateral margins
and tip of the tongue. These heal without scarring.

   These clinical features are almost always sufficient to allow
of a diagnosis after proper examination and history taking.
Biopsy is unproductive except in the occasional situation in
which a long standing major aphthous ulcer is suspected of malignancy. Any of these three varieties of R.O.U. may be associated
with lesions of the eyes or of the genital or perianal structures.
This triad is usually referred to as Behçet's syndrome although,
in fact, the fully developed syndrome is a widespread condition
involving auto-immune damage to many structures including the
central nervous system and joints and blood vessels.

   In a certain number of patients R.O.U. is associated with
coeliac disease and the treatment of this by the adoption of a
gluten free diet leads to a cessation of the ulceration. The
association with haematological and nutritional disturbances has
not yet been fully explored but there is no doubt that such
associations do exist. In view of these facts supplementary
investigations should include a full blood count, serum iron,
folate and B_{12} estimations. If an abnormality is shown (particularly a depressed serum iron or folate level) then the patient
should be considered for jejeunal biopsy to eliminate the possibility of coeliac disease.

For summary see Table VII, p97.

Bullous Lesions
   A bulla is simply a blister and there is no real difference
between the meaning of this term and that of the term 'vesicle'.
However, 'bulla' is usually used in the context of larger
blisters whereas 'vesicle' is most commonly used to describe
multiple small blisters.

   The important bullous diseases which produce lesions in the
mouth are three in number (pemphigus, pemphigoid and benign
mucous membrane pemphigoid) although some other conditions - such
as dermatitis herpetiformis - occasionally produce bullae within
the mouth. Occasionally also, lichen planus undergoes a transient bullous phase and blisters may be seen on the oral mucosa.
A more permanent condition of bullous lichen planus is, however,
far less common than was at one time suggested. These unusual
presentations must evidently be kept in mind but for the purposes
of the present discussion the three more common conditions are
considered.

TABLE VII

RECURRENT ORAL ULCERATION - SUMMARY

MINOR APHTHOUS ULCERS

1 - 6 at a time.
2 - 10 mm diameter, non-indurated.
Last 10 days - variable interval.
Not in throat or palate.
Heal without scarring.

MAJOR APHTHOUS ULCERS

Variable number at a time -
usually few.
May be very large, indurated.
May last months, variable
interval.
Affect palate and oro-pharynx.
Heal with scarring or tissue
destruction.

Differential diagnosis - from
carcinoma, major erosive lichen
planus.

HERPETIFORM ULCERS

Large number of very small
painful ulcers.
Occasionally coalesce to form
larger ulcers.
Variable duration - about 2 weeks.
Variable interval usually months.
Typically floor of mouth, margins
of tongue.

Differential diagnosis - from
herpes, other viral infections.

INVESTIGATIONS

F.B.C., Serum iron, T.I.B.C.,
Saturation, Folate, B_{12}.

Jejeunal biopsy if indicated.

Pemphigus. Pemphigus is a chronic disorder of skin and
mucous membranes marked by acantholysis and the consequent separation of the epithelium above the basal cell layer. This,
followed by oedema into the tissue cleft, produces fluid filled
bullae which eventually rupture. These lesions are often first
found in the mouth, most commonly on the palatal mucosa, but
eventually spread over a considerable area of the body. Previously to the introduction of steroids and antibiotics, secondary
infection and debility frequently led to a fatal conclusion but
there is now some degree of control. Since the first lesions are
often oral bullae alone - apparently before the onset of skin
lesions or of any significant malaise - it is important that an
accurate diagnosis should be made at this stage.

The patients are predominantly in the 40 to 60 year old age
group at the time of the first lesions and there is a high incidence in Jewish patients. The lesions in the mouth present as
thin walled fluid filled vesicles up to 1 cm in diameter. These
rapidly break down and at this stage the covering epithelium is
seen in shreds attached at the margin of the lesion. Secondary
infection follows and the lesion is converted to a painful ulcer.
Skin lesions are usually larger - up to several centimetres in
diameter - and the process of breakdown and secondary infection
occurs less rapidly. Nikolsky's sign is positive, the epithelial
layer being easily wiped off the oral mucosa.

Initial diagnosis is by recognition of the acantholytic cells
of the epithelium. Fluid from the bullae or scrapings from the
lesions show the typical rounded hyperchromic cells of acantholysis (Fig. 3.1). Smear biopsy should be supplemented by excisional biopsy of an early lesion if possible. Because of the
fragility of the bullae this may be a difficult procedure. If
electron microscopic facilities are available characteristic
changes in the epithelium may be seen and confirm the diagnosis.

The most important modern diagnostic aid to differentiate
between the bullous diseases is immunofluorescence. Patients
with pemphigus have autoantibodies active against the prickle
cell layer of the epithelium and these are highly specific. Both
direct and indirect immunofluorescent techniques may be used to
detect these antibodies (Fig. 2.6).

Pemphigoid. Pemphigoid is a result of blistering occurring
from below the basal cell layer of the epithelium which is
lifted intact by the fluid. As a result of this the bullae, both
of skin and mucous membrane, are relatively firm. There is no
acantholysis and, therefore, no acantholytic cells in the bulla
fluid. In contrast to pemphigus the oral mucosa is affected in
only 20% of patients. There is no racial susceptibility and most
patients are over the age of sixty years. Like pemphigus, pemphigoid is a disease both of skin and mucous membrane - this is in
contrast to benign mucous membrane pemphigoid which is more common
and is almost completely restricted to the mucous membranes.

The diagnostic techniques applied to pemphigoid are similar to
those for pemphigus. Cytological examination of bulla fluid,

biopsy and immunofluorescent techniques are all used to confirm
the clinical diagnosis. In the case of pemphigoid, antibody
deposition is at the basement membrane and not within the prickle
cell layer.

Benign mucous membrane pemphigoid In this condition most
patients are female and are over the age of sixty years. Again
there is no racial prevalence. The condition presents as bullae
of mucous membranes which rupture and heal with some degree of
scar formation. Skin bullae rarely appear. Most commonly the
soft palate is involved - the area is likely to remain restricted
rather than to spread. However, the conjunctival sac is an
important further site for bulla formation followed by scarring,
and if the condition is allowed to progress this may lead to loss
of sight. It is therefore particularly important that attention
be paid to initial eye signs and symptoms in patients with this
condition.

The diagnostic techniques are as outlined for the other bullous conditions. As in pemphigoid, antibodies are found at the
level of the basement membrane.

For summary see Table VIII (p100)

Acute Vesicular Conditions
     There are two relatively common acute conditions in which
multiple vesicles occur on the oral mucous membrane. These are
acute herpetic stomatitis and erythema multiforme. Although the
aetiologies of these two conditions are quite different there
may be considerable similarities between their clinical presentation and differential diagnosis may be difficult. There is,
however, one factor of absolute diagnostic significance - acute
herpetic stomatitis is invariably a primary lesion only and does
not recur. Erythema multiforme on the other hand is characteristically a recurrent condition.

Acute herpetic stomatitis. This represents the primary infection by the herpes simplex virus and usually occurs in early life
- between the ages of one and six years. If adulthood has been
reached without herpetic infection this primary lesion may occur
at any time, although predominantly in young adults. There is
often a history of recent contact with a patient suffering from
recurrent facial herpes (cold sores).

The first stage in the condition is the onset of malaise and
fever together with submandibular lymphadenitis. This early
lymph node involvement is an important diagnostic feature. It is
rapidly followed by the development of vesicles which may be any-
where on the oral mucosa. These rapidly break down to form
ulcers which may extend on to the external vermilion border of
the lip. There may also be vesicular eruptions on the skin
around the mouth although the condition is mainly confined to the
mucosa. The mouth is extremely sore and stagnation may occur
with a non-specific halitosis. In young children a marked gingivitis is common, the gingival margins being red and swollen and

TABLE VIII

BULLOUS LESIONS - SUMMARY

PEMPHIGUS
Age 40 - 60, F:M - 1:1
Fragile bullae, early in mouth
Skin & mucous membranes
Jewish patients +
Histology - acantholysis, intra-epithelial bulla
Immunoglobulins in prickle cell layer.

PEMPHIGOID
Age 60+, F:M - 1:1
Tough bullae
Skin & mucous membranes
No racial prevalence
Histology - no acantholysis, subepithelial bulla
Immunoglobulins at basement membrane

BENIGN MUCOUS MEMBRANE PEMPHIGOID
Age 60+, F:M - 2:1
Bullae often on soft palate
Later involvement of conjunctivae
Heals with scar formation
Histology - no acantholysis, subepithelial bulla
Immunoglobulins at basement membrane

OTHER BULLOUS LESIONS
  DERMATITIS HERPETIFORMIS,
  BULLOUS LICHEN PLANUS,
  EPIDERMOLYSIS BULLOSA,
  DRUG REACTIONS
Rare, but to be considered in differential diagnosis.

occasionally bleeding. The clinical condition in the child,
apart from its sudden onset, is reminiscent of that in acute
leukaemia. It is unusual for the gingivitis to be such a prominent symptom in the adult patient. After approximately a week of
pain and discomfort the condition resolves by gradual subsidence
over some 3-4 further days. This resolution is not by elimination of the virus, which remains in the tissues. Later symptoms,
however, are much less severe and are restricted to the typical
"cold sores" at or about the mucocutaneous junction which appear
when there is some slightly debilitating condition. These recurrent facial lesions follow in approximately half the patients.

Diagnosis of primary herpes is from the clinical picture in
the first instance. Confirmation is given by the presence of
viral inclusion bodies and other abnormalities in the epithelial
cells taken by smear techniques from the vicinity of the ulcers
(Fig. 3.3). Specific antiviral antibodies are produced after a
few days and increase to a maximum in 14 days. This rise in
antibodies is demonstrated by determining the increase in the
titre at an interval of 10 days - so long as the first titre is
taken at an early stage a significant rise is diagnostic. If
animal host or tissue culture techniques are available these may
be used to confirm the nature of the virus although direct electron microscopy, when available, is faster and accurate (Fig. 3.4).

Erythema multiforme. This is a recurrent acute vesicular
condition predominantly affecting the oral mucosa in a manner
closely resembling acute herpetic stomatitis; however, the
condition is characteristically recurrent. The precise aetiology
of the condition is not known although it is thought to be of
auto-immune origin. In a typical attack vesicles may form on the
whole of the oral mucosa, but in particular on the lower lip.
These vesicles rapidly break down to form crusting ulcers, the
lip again being prominently affected. Submandibular lymph node
involvement may occur but usually at a somewhat later stage than
in acute herpetic stomatitis. Associated skin lesions may occur
in typical 'target' form and these also provide confirmatory
diagnosis of the oral condition. A widespread form of this condition, with marked involvement of large areas of skin and of
other mucous membranes, is known as the Stevens-Johnson syndrome.
There is, however, no real difference between the two conditions
- merely one of extent and severity. Attacks of erythema multiforme may be precipitated by a number of agencies, a fact which
may complicate diagnosis. Viral or bacterial infections, the
presence of neoplasms, pregnancy and a wide variety of drug reactions have all been implicated. Of these recurrent herpes
simplex is probably the most common precipitating factor.

As pointed out above, laboratory investigations are not particularly productive in cases of erythema multiforme. Biopsy is
occasionally carried out in the case of doubtful early lesions
and this may be helpful. Urine analysis not infrequently shows
the presence of protein during an attack which is apparently
otherwise restricted to the mouth - presumably this indicates
the presence of genito-urinary mucosal involvement. A mild
eosinophilia may be seen in the blood film but otherwise haemat-

ological changes tend to be associated with secondary factors -
particularly infection. Characteristic electron microscopic
appearances have been described and may be occasionally of value
in diagnosis in doubtful cases and if facilities are available.

Coxsackie virus infections. Relatively mild infections by the
coxsackie viruses occur in humans. Herpangina is caused by the
A4 type virus and hand-foot-mouth disease by the A16 type.

Herpangina is a mild infection which is often seen in mild
epidemic form amongst children. The patients complain of a sore
throat and a certain degree of general malaise. Rather non-
specific small vesicles appear at the back of the mouth and the
oro-pharynx and last for five days or so before resolving. The
lesions have no particular characteristic appearance and resemble
other lesions of viral origin. However, their distribution at
the back of the mouth and, in particular, in the soft palate, is
a diagnostic indicator.

In hand-foot-mouth disease vesicles may appear widely distributed over the oral mucosa. They are associated with a vesicular
rash on the palms of the hands and the soles of the feet. The
oral vesicles rapidly break down and may be observed predominantly as ulcers. As in herpangina, the generalised symptoms are
minor and the symptoms resolve after about five days. This is
not the same condition as foot and mouth disease which is much
more severe and caused by a quite different virus.

Herpes zoster. Two clinical conditions appear in humans as a
result of infection by herpes zoster virus - chicken pox and
herpes zoster - although it has never been proved that the two
conditions can be mutually infective. In herpes zoster a vesicular eruption occurs, typically restricted to the peripheral
distribution of a sensory nerve. In the facial area the eruption
commonly attacks the distribution of the opthalmic division of
the trigeminal nerve and the eye may be severely affected. On
the skin there is an early phase of pain and tenderness which is
followed by the production of a vesicular rash. Within the oral
cavity the lesions appear much as those of herpes simplex and,
although the restriction to a particular nerve distribution may
give an indication as to the nature of the infection this is not
a reliable guide - herpes simplex may also occur in a restricted
distribution of this kind. The lesions of herpes zoster fade
over a relatively long time and there is often considerable
systemic upset. A most important eventual complication is post
herpetic neuralgia occurring in the area of the rash.

Diagnosis of infections by the coxsackie viruses and by
herpes zoster can be confirmed by the methods outlined in Chapter III and similar to those used for the identification of
herpes simplex. In view of the mildness of the condition it is
probably true that many infections due to the coxsackie virus
pass undiagnosed. In the case of herpes zoster, however, the
severity of the initial and consequential symptoms is such as to
call for full viral identification studies. For summary see
Table IX (p103).

TABLE IX

ACUTE VESICULAR LESIONS - SUMMARY

ACUTE HERPETIC STOMATITIS   Non recurrent. Children, young
                              adults.
                              Mouth and lips. Gingivitis
                              (especially children).
                              History of contact with recurrent
                              herpes.
                              Viral tests positive (rising
                              antibody titre, inclusion bodies,
                              direct electron microscopy) for
                              Herpes hominis 1.

ERYTHEMA MULTIFORME   Recurrent. Young adults.
                              Mouth and lips (especially lower
                              lip).
                              Skin lesions ('target')
                              Viral tests negative (but may be
                              precipitated by herpes).

HERPES ZOSTER   Non recurrent. Adults.
                              Localised distribution on skin or
                              mucous membrane.
                              Painful vesicular rash. Severe
                              malaise.
                              Viral tests positive.

HERPANGINA   Mild infection. Predominantly
                              children.
                              Vesicles posterior part of mouth.
                              Often in epidemic form.
                              Viral tests positive (Coxsackie
                              A4)

HAND-FOOT-MOUTH   Mild infection.
                              Vesicles mouth, palms and soles.
                              Viral tests positive (Coxsackie
                              A16).

White Patches

Lesions which form white patches on the oral mucous membrane
may be classified for diagnostic purposes in three broad groups:

1. Lesions in which superficial white plaques
    form over the epithelial surface. The
    predominant condition of this kind is acute
    pseudomembranous candidiasis (thrush).

2. Intrinsic white patches of the oral mucosa
    itself caused by identifiable agencies such
    as trauma or chemical burns.

3. Intrinsic white patches of the oral mucosa
    with no evident local causative factor.

The diagnostic significance of candidiasis will be dealt with
in a later section. Lesions in group 2 (those with identifiable
local causative agents) may be considered as follows:-

Traumatic keratosis. Mechanical irritation of the mucosa may
cause the production of lesions varying from acute ulceration to
a white patch - the so-called traumatic keratosis. Generally
this latter is produced by long term irritation of a relatively
low grade. The most usual site is along the occlusal level of
the buccal mucosa but lesions are also common on unprotected
edentulous alveolar mucosa. The diagnosis is almost entirely
clinical and largely depends on recognition of the irritant factor. It is evident that if suspicion of a sinister change is
aroused by the form of the lesion or if it continues to progress
after the removal of the irritant cause then confirmation by
biopsy is essential.

Chemical burns. These usually follow the use of aspirin or an
aspirin containing mixture as a local application for toothache.
The lesion may be thick and densely white, often surrounded by an
erythematous area. Its diagnosis is again entirely clinical,
depending on the history of acute onset, the presence of the
offending tooth and the confirmatory history by the patient.
Similar lesions following dental treatment may be due to the use
of substances such as root treatment medicaments.

Tobacco induced lesions. The relationship between the use of
tobacco and the formation of white lesions on the oral mucosa is
unclear. There seems good evidence that many cases classified as
leukoplakia may have at least a partial aetiology of this kind.
It is, however, very difficult to state without question that a
specific lesion is due to the use of tobacco in any of its forms.
An exception to this statement is the pipe-smoker's palate. This
lesion almost, but not entirely, confined to the smokers of pipe
tobacco, has a quite characteristic clinical appearance. A diffuse white lesion occurs across the palate accompanied by swelling of the mucous glands. A polygonal 'crazy paving' pattern is
thus provided in the centre of each small section being the dila-
ted duct of a mucous gland. This pattern is usually most marked
at the posterior part of the hard palate. Diagnosis can usually

be made with some confidence on a clinical basis although quite
clearly, if abnormal characteristics appear, biopsy is essential.

   Leukoplakia. A wide range of generalised conditions may result in the production of white patches of the oral mucosa, the
most common of these being lichen planus. With the exception of
this, however, the great majority of white patches on the oral
mucosa are isolated to that site.

The term 'leukoplakia' (which evidently also means white
patch) has acquired a specialised meaning. In the past it was
used to imply premalignancy and is still occasionally considered
in this way. However, it is now general to accept the clinical
definition put forward by Pindborg - "a white patch on the oral
mucosa which cannot be wiped away and is not susceptible to any
other clinical diagnosis". Included within the definition are a
range of lesions which vary in their clinical aggresiveness from
almost entirely benign to incipiently malignant - the differentiation within this group is entirely by biopsy and histological
assessment.

There are a number of variations in the appearance of leukoplakias and recognition of these is particularly important since
they can to some degree be related to the prognosis of the lesions. Homogenous leukoplakia, as the name implies, consists of
a relatively uniformly white patch sometimes with folding and
fissuring of the surface. In speckled leukoplakia white patches
appear on a red background. These speckled lesions, often associated with candidal infection, are considered to have a higher
degree of premalignant potential than homogenous leukoplakias.
Erythroplakia consists of a red velvety patch of the mucosa,
often (but not invariably) associated with surrounding white
areas. In such a lesion the epithelium is atrophic but contains
many epithelial atypia - this is a particularly sinister lesion.
Preleukoplakia is the term used to describe an early lesion of
the mucosa in which a faint greyish patch represents a halfway
stage to the formation of a leukoplakia proper. In all these
cases a definitive final diagnosis depends on the taking of a
biopsy specimen of the incisional or excisional type - smear biopsy is virtually useless.

   Histological assessment. In the past, histological assessment
of potentially malignant lesions has depended entirely on subjective study. This, however, is difficult and the number of methods designed to include a degree of objective assessment have
been introduced. These depend largely on the adoption of scoring
techniques for various criteria of abnormality in order to produce an index which it is hoped will indicate eventual clinical
behaviour. The production of data in a digital form also allows
of a more objective analysis of results and preliminary experi-
ments have been carried out using computer analyses of such data.
Initial results seem to be highly encouraging. A future development might well include the electronic scanning of tissue for
abnormality - a technique which is now available in the case of
uterine cervical smears.

The investigation of white patches on the oral mucosa depends
on observation of the following points:-

1. A careful medical history, including
   details of any skin complaints from
   which the patient may suffer or has
   suffered in the past.

2. Elimination of the possibility of
   genetically determined lesions (these
   are, in fact, very rare).

3. The elimination of the possibility of
   oral lesions of dermatological disease
   - in particular of lichen planus. This
   differentiation may depend entirely on
   the biopsy although in some instances
   (e.g. reticular lichen planus) the clinical
   pattern may be characteristic. Lesions
   may be confined to the mouth.

4. The elimination of local mucosal irritants,
   either mechanical (such as broken teeth or
   sharp edged fillings) or from the use of
   tobacco.

5. Haematological screening tests may be of
   help in some circumstances. In particular
   the carrying out of serological tests for
   syphilis is often recommended as a routine
   in cases of white lesions of unknown origin.
   In European conditions the association
   between leukoplakia and syphilis is now an
   uncommon one although in other societies
   this is not necessarily the case.

6. Swabs and smears (especially in superficial
   lesions).

7. Biopsy - in many cases the most significant
   form of investigation.

N.B. There is always the possibility that an apparently
     simple white lesion may prove to be a carcinoma.
     Only biopsy can determine this.

Candidiasis
    Candida albicans is present in the mouths of most healthy
individuals, maintaining a commensal balance with the host. When
this balance is disturbed by a loss of the patient's protective
mechanisms a clinical infection takes place. Candidiasis - and
in particular acute pseudomembranous candidiasis - is therefore a
condition which occurs in tissues already weakened in some way by
a generalised disturbance or by localised trauma. The investigation of a patient with such a condition implies a double responsibility - firstly to make the initial diagnosis of candidiasis
and secondly to identify the underlying reason for its presence.
Oral candidiasis may be classified under four headings (angular
cheilitis, with candida as the infective organism, may be associated with any of these four).

    Acute pseudomembranous candidiasis (Thrush). The candidal
infection is superficial, the organisms proliferating to form a
plaque in which is incorporated debris of various kinds, including bacteria and desquamated epithelial cells. This plaque can
be wiped away leaving a raw bleeding surface behind. Direct
identification of the condition is easily carried out by making a
direct smear from such a scraping. This, stained preferably with
PAS stain, shows the mass of tangled hyphae characteristic of the
infection. (See Chapter III).

    Acute atrophic candidiasis. In this form of candidiasis the
atrophic mucosa is painful and bright red. The organisms do not
form a membrane of the surface but penetrate within the tissues.
A scraping is therefore much less productive of organisms than in
the case of thrush, although some are usually to be seen. Acute
atrophic candidiasis is perhaps most often seen in patients in
whom the immune response is supressed by the use of systemic
steroids or in whom the balance of oral flora is disturbed by the
taking of wide spectrum antibiotics. The 'antibiotic sore
tongue' is an example of this condition.

    Chronic atrophic candidiasis. This, in the form of denture
sore mouth, is the most common form of oral candidiasis. The
picture of painless erythema of the palate, restricted to the
area covered by the dentures, is quite characteristic. Again
swabs from the surface may not produce a great deal of evidence
of candidal infection - swabs from the fitting surface of the
denture however are likely to be much more productive. Denture
sore mouth is not generally associated with ill health and only
in unusually persistent or severe cases is it considered necessary to screen the patient for abnormality. However, the appearance of diffuse chronic atrophic candidosis in the absence of a
denture is very occasionally a sign of endocrine disturbances
as, for instance, in Addison's disease.

    Chronic hyperplastic candidiasis. This condition is also
known as candidal leukoplakia and has been briefly considered
above. The clinical presentation may be identical with other
leukoplakias and its diagnosis is almost entirely histological,
depending on the staining of sections with PAS to identify the
organisms within the epithelium. This is a significant condition

since the presence of candida in such lesions is generally considered to be a sign of increased premalignant potential.

For summary of candidiasis see Table X p109.

Lichen Planus

Lichen planus warrants separate consideration as being the
skin disease in which oral lesions are most often seen.   The
skin lesions appear as dusky pink papules, often with white
streaks on the surface - these are known as Wickham's striae.
The skin lesions may be distributed over a number of sites but
most commonly occur on the flexor surfaces of the wrists, a convenient site for examination in the dental clinic.   The skin
lesions may produce irritation and itching, but this is variable.
Approximately 70% of patients with skin lesions also have lesions
of the oral mucosa.   It does not follow that the same percentage
of patients with oral lesions also have skin lesions - the equivalent percentage is of the order of 30-40%.   The reason for this
variation is probably the fact that the oral lesions are in many
cases asymptomatic and may occur at a different time from the
skin lesions - it is believed that many patients with oral lesions may have had transient minor skin lesions previously.   The
patients with oral lesions of lichen planus are predominantly
female (70%) and with a wide age range.

The essential changes in lichen planus consist of the laying
down of a well defined band of inflammatory cells (predominantly
lymphocytes) in the connective tissue below the basement membrane.   Above this the epithelium may undergo a wide range of
changes, from hyperparakeratinisation on the one hand to atrophy
on the other.   This variety of histological changes in the epithelium corresponds to an equally wide range of clinical presentations which may make initial diagnosis difficult.   However, the
histological appearances are usually characteristic and simple
biopsy examination most often leads to a definite diagnosis -
complex techniques (such as immunofluorescence) are not required.

Although a number of possible alternative classifications of
the clinical variants of lichen planus exist, a simple scheme,
based on the clinical features, is a division into three groups
1) non-erosive lichen planus 2) minor erosive lichen planus and
3) major erosive lichen planus.

Non-erosive lichen planus.   In this form the histological
changes are of hyperparakeratosis or hyperorthokeratosis of the
epithelium reflected in the clinical appearance of a white
lesion without ulceration.   These lesions may present as white
striations arranged in a reticular pattern over the mucosa.
These are thought to be similar to the Wickham's striae appearing
on the skin lesions.   In many patients, however, this classical
appearance of reticulation does not occur and the lesions may
have a papular or confluent appearance which may lead to a clinical diagnosis of leukoplakia.   These non-erosive lesions are
virtually symptomless and are often first noted accidentally by
the patient or dental surgeon.

TABLE X

CANDIDIASIS - SUMMARY

ACUTE PSEUDOMEMBRANOUS   White superficial patches.
        ('Thrush')   Wipes off, leaving bleeding
                               area.
                               Candida + in smears.
                               Investigate for systemic
                               condition (blood, urine etc.)

ACUTE ATROPHIC   Red painful mucosa.
                               Few candida in smears.
                               Patient often on steroids,
                               antibiotics.
                               (e.g. 'antibiotic sore tongue')

CHRONIC ATROPHIC   Usually 'denture sore mouth'
                               Painless red area below upper
                               denture.
                               Few candida on palatal smears,
                               more on denture.
                               Diagnosis clinical, full
                               screening not usually required.

CHRONIC HYPERPLASTIC   White patches - intrinsic.
                               Few organisms on smears.
                               Diagnosis - histology (P.A.S.
                               stain)

Any of the above oral conditions may be associated with

        (a) angular cheilitis
        (b) candidiasis of skin, nails etc. -
            in systemic disease (especially
            immune deficiencies) and immuno
            supression.

<u>Minor erosive lichen planus</u>. In this form of oral lichen
planus the predominating histological change is of atrophy of
the epithelium. This corresponds to the clinically evident
erosions caused by disintegration and loss of the weakened
atrophic epithelial layer. The areas of erosion are often associated with other non-erosive areas of lichen planus, the whole
presenting a fairly distinctive picture. However, there are a
number of possible differential diagnoses and confirmation must
be carried out by biopsy examination. In this variant of lichen
planus there is often considerable discomfort.

<u>Major erosive lichen planus</u>. In this variant of oral lichen
planus the lesions consist essentially of large ulcers of the
mucosa, the result of widespread breakdown of the weakened
epithelium. The onset is usually acute and is most common in
older patients. Although the predominant lesion is of ulceration there are almost always some areas of whiteness which give
a clue to the essential nature of the condition. Biopsy of
these areas confirms the histology of lichen planus.

Lichen planus is not usually associated with any other generalised condition but it has recently been suggested that there
may be an association with maturity onset diabetes or hyper-
tension in some patients. These suggestions have not been confirmed by further work and the association should, at the present
time, be considered as unproven. It should be remembered that,
if it is decided to test for latent maturity onset diabetes, a
urine test may not be helpful. A glucose tolerance test is necessary to fully eliminate the possibility of latent diabetes
(Chapter II). It should also be noted that lichen planus may
appear as a response to drugs. This, the so called 'lichenoid
reaction', is indistinguishable from the non drug induced form.

Diffuse Stomatitis
A number of patients present with the complaint of a generalised soreness of the mouth, often particularly affecting the
tongue. This may be associated with a sensation of dryness of
the mouth or of alterations in taste sensation, although the
patient may show no obvious changes in the oral mucosa or in
salivary flow. The assessment of these patients is carried out
on the following lines:-

1. The elimination of any evident and recognisable
    lesion (such as geographic tongue, lichen
    planus etc.).

2. The elimination of any possible mechanical
    irritating factor, for example, new dentures.
    A change of tobacco using habit may also be of
    importance.

3. The elimination of a drug induced stomatitis.
    A wide range of medications may be responsible,
    including the antirheumatic drugs and steroids.
    (See also Chapter IX).

4. Tests for haematological abnormalities.

5. Urine analysis for the presence of glucose.
    In cases of doubt a blood sugar estimation
    and glucose tolerance test should be carried
    out.

6. Assessment of salivary flow and salivary gland
    function may be carried out (see Chapter IX).

Not all patients need such a comprehensive scheme of investigation and, in particular, the assessment of salivary gland function is one not to be undertaken lightly.

A full haematological investigation for the present purposes
would consist of the following investigations and estimations:-
full blood count and film, haemoglobin, serum iron, total iron
binding capacity, saturation, serum B_{12}, folate, erythrocyte
sedimentation rate.

Haematological abnormalities of various kinds may give rise to
a wide range of oral changes, most of which are non-specific to
any basic aetiology. Those most commonly associated with anaemias, latent anaemias and similar disturbances are sore tongue,
generalised stomatitis, taste disturbance, ulceration, candidiasis
and angular cheilitis. Such changes, or the onset of generalised
soreness in an apparently normal oral mucosa, may be the earliest
indication of the haematological disturbance. Perhaps the most
sensitive indicator of these changes is the state of papillation
of the tongue.

Objective measurement of disturbances in the sense of taste
are very difficult to carry out and rarely form part of the
examination in such cases. In investigating such a patient some
possible aetiological factors for the complaint of abnormality of
taste should be borne in mind:-

1. Recent insertion of a prosthetic appliance of some
    kind.

2. The presence of infection in the mouth or related
    structures.

3. A side effect of drugs.

4. Early pernicious anaemia. The disturbance in taste
    sensation may occur before any other signs or symp-
    toms have become evident.

5. Lesions of the central nervous system (very rare).

However, many patients complaining of abnormalities of taste
are never at any time shown to have any physical abnormality.
Some of the commoner manifestations of diffuse stomatitis and
their causative factors are shown in Table XI.

TABLE XI

DIFFUSE NON SPECIFIC STOMATITIS AND GLOSSITIS

Causative factors - summary

MECHANICAL TRAUMA

IRON DEFICIENCY (anaemia or latent anaemia)

FOLATE DEFICIENCY

B_{12} DEFICIENCY (e.g. early pernicious anaemia)

TOBACCO

DIABETES MELLITUS

POOR SALIVARY FLOW (e.g. in Sjögren's Syndrome)

CANDIDIASIS (secondary to some other factor)

ENDOCRINE DISTURBANCES

INCIPIENT LICHEN PLANUS

DRUG INDUCED

Neoplasia

Neoplasms, benign or malignant, primary or secondary and of all types may occur in the mouth. Although there are sites of predilection, typical forms and recognizable textures, the final diagnosis must depend entirely on biopsy.

The question of incisional versus excisional biopsy depends largely on the size of the suspect lesion. If small, and if a reasonable margin of apparently normal tissue may be removed around and below the lesion, then excisional biopsy is best even though the margins of apparently normal tissue removed may be much less than might have to be removed should the lesion in fact turn out to be malignant.

An exception to this generalization is in the case of the malignant melanoma. Melanoma of the oral cavity is rare but highly malignant and any hope of cure depends on early diagnosis. The lesion occurs usually in middle life and is most frequently found on the alveolar and palatal mucosa. In its early stages the lesion presents as a black patch on the mucosa often without any induration or ulceration. Such a melanotic patch should invariably be excised for biopsy purposes together with a margin of apparently normal tissue. Incisional biopsy, by causing dissemination of malignant cells may, in this instance, make a poor prognosis even worse.

Carcinoma. Carcinoma may present, particularly in the early stages, in forms which are entirely non-classical. Rolled-edged indurated ulcers, proliferative growths and similar lesions are immediately suspect, but it is the lesion which stimulates in its early stages a simple keratosis, a simple ulcer or even a mild erythema which it is most vital to diagnose and to allow of treatment at the optimum time. The two points which justify re-emphasis are that the malignant lesion may show none of the expected typical malignant signs and that it is impossible clinically to differentiate between leukoplakia and frank malignancy in the marginal case.

Thus, biopsy is mandatory in every case in which the slightest possibility of carcinoma arises - any ulcer not healed within 10 days or any white area or erythema which is not obvious in its aetiology. As has been explained in Chapter III, smear biopsy is insufficient for final diagnosis. Incisional or excisional biopsy is indicated in all cases in which sufficient doubt arises to carry out investigation at all. The simplicity of the technique, the availability of the site and the reliability of the diagnosis thereby obtained demands tissue examination. The situation in respect of mouth cancer is quite different from that of uterine cervical lesions in which smear biopsy has proved successful as a screening test for malignancy. Biopsy in the mouth is not carried out as a screening test but for the investigation of some specific lesion and, this being the case, maximum information must be gained at the first investigation.

It should always be remembered that a diagnosis of carcinoma

should be followed as closely as possible by treatment and it is
imperative that anyone who is prepared to biopsy a suspect lesion
should be prepared to arrange for immediate treatment if necessary.

Lymph node enlargement in oral carcinoma occurs relatively
early. The location of involved nodes depends on the lymphatic
pathways from the lesion which may become blocked by malignant
emboli and form collateral drainage routes. Thus bilateral and
other apparently unanatomical lymph node swelling may occur.
This swelling does not indicate necessarily metastatic growth.
The early lymph node swelling is in response to some nonspecific
inflammatory reaction which may be increased by secondary infection in the neoplasm. This lymphadenitis may occur well before
metastatic deposits are laid down. Thus examination of the lymph
nodes of the head and neck must be carried out in any case of
suspected malignancy, with these factors in mind.

Pigmentation of the Oral Mucosa
Pigmentation of the oral mucosa may occur in a variety of
situations, both physiological and pathological.

Normal variations. There is a wide range of normal patterns
of melanotic pigmentation. Most races with heavily pigmented
skins also have considerable pigmentation of the oral mucosa
which may be patchy in distribution and which almost always invol-
ves the gingivae. Such pigmentation may also occur in an irregular manner in individuals with less pigmented skins. This represents an entirely normal situation.

Increased melanotic pigmentation. An established marked
increase in melanotic pigmentation in the oral mucosa may be associated with generalised disease. Of these the most usual is
Addison's disease in which increased activity of the melanocytes
is stimulated by the endocrine upset of the condition. The pigmentation may occur on the buccal mucosa, palate, or on any other
area of the oral mucosa and may appear early in the disease.
Other signs of endocrine dysfunction (such as malaise, lowering
of the blood pressure and weight loss) together with a bronzed
appearance of the skin also caused by increased melanocyte activity, soon follow. It is important to realise that the presence of
melanotic pigmentation on the oral mucosa in itself does not call
for a full endocrine investigation, it is the increase in melanotic pigmentation or its incidence where none was previously
present which should cause concern. Further investigation of
such patients should be in the hands of the endocrinologist,
rather than the dental surgeon, if it is considered justified.

In inflammatory conditions. In some inflammatory and similar
conditions of the oral mucosa (in particular oral lichen planus)
increased melanotic pigmentation may occur and this may be evident both clinically and histologically. In itself this pigmentation is of no clinical significance and does not warrant further investigation.

Naevae and melanomas. Small benign melanotic patches may
occasionally appear on the oral mucosa and cause concern. In the
early stages of malignant melanoma formation it may be difficult
to distinguish the lesion from an innocent one, and this may be
done only by biopsy according to the methods outlined above. In
general any pigmented area of recent origin which is sufficiently
suspicious to justify biopsy should be treated by these methods
i.e. wide excision biopsy.

Amalgam pigmentation. Pigmentation of the oral mucosa by
ectopic amalgam is common. The particles of amalgam are generally visible on x-ray but, after a period of time, the metallic
element may become widely distributed in the tissues and so not
visible on x-ray. The site of the pigmented patch (practically
always on the gingivae and in relation to a filled tooth) may
give a strong clue as to the nature of the colouration but in
rare instances the site may be, for various reasons, quite atypical.

Drug induced pigmentation. A wide range of drugs have been
implicated in the production of pigmentation of the oral mucosa.
A careful drug history is therefore of great importance in investigation of an unusual pigmentation. Formerly the heavy metals
were most often implicated in this kind of pigmentation, (for
instance the classical gingival lead line). At the present time,
however, the pigmentation induced by drugs is most commonly due
to the use of anti-malarials or tranquillizers. Oral pigmentation
is also a side effect attributed to the use of oral contraceptives.

Vascular lesions simulating melanotic patches. It is important
to recognize that a patch of melanotic pigmentation may be simul-
ated by the presence of a vascular abnormality in the mucous membrane. In most cases it is possible to differentiate by pressing
gently on the suspect area with a glass slide. In the case of a
blood filled vascular lesion the emptying of the underlying vessels is easily seen, whereas the structure of a melanotic lesion
is equally evident.

The causes of oral melanotic pigmentation are summarised in
Table XII.

Fibro-epithelial polyp. This common lesion, consisting of
scar tissue, presents as a pedunculated or sessile spherical firm
swelling of the mucosa - most commonly the buccal mucosa. It is
related to some point of trauma - often on the occlusal plane.
The lesion is completely symptom free unless traumatized and may
grow undisturbed from its usual size at diagnosis - approximately
1 cm in diameter - to a remarkably large size. The texture of
the lesion reflects its histological composition, varying from
soft immature fibrous tissue to tough and partly calcified tissue
in the case of very large longstanding lesions. The colour is
pale pink. Diagnosis is by appearance, by its clear relation to
a source of trauma and by histological confirmation following
excision.

Denture granuloma. This lesion is essentially the same as the fibro-epithelial polyp, the irritating factor being the margin of an ill-fitting denture. Because of its relation to the denture the lesion tends to be elongated and is often folded to enclose the denture flange. It is quite painless unless secondary ulceration occurs. Diagnosis, as in the case of the polyp, is by appearance, by its relation to the denture periphery, and by confirmatory histological investigation.

TABLE XII

PIGMENTATION OF THE ORAL MUCOSA - SUMMARY

NORMAL MELANOTIC PIGMENTATION - of ethnic origin.

ABNORMAL MELANOTIC PIGMENTATION (i.e. increased
    melanin production) - usually in endocrine
    disturbances.

SECONDARY MELANIN PRODUCTION IN INFLAMMATORY AND
    SIMILAR LESIONS - e.g. lichen planus,
    leukoplakia.

NAEVAE AND MELANOMAS.

AMALGAM PIGMENTATION.

DRUG INDUCED PIGMENTATION (formerly heavy metals:
    Now anti-malarials, tranquillizers, oral
    contraceptives).

Chapter VII

Lesions of Bone: Cysts

Inflammatory Lesions of Bone

Osteomyelitis

Osteomyelitis - inflammatory changes in the soft tissue components of the bones with secondary changes in the calcified tissues - occurs in the jawbones in two clinical variants according
to the age of the patient, although there is no real difference
between the basic pathological processes.

In the adult the condition occurs much more commonly in the
mandible by direct extension of some odontogenic infection. A
wide variety of causative organisms has been identified and no
specific organism has been predominantly implicated. The acute
form is often heralded by some readily identifiable local focus
of infection such as an alveolar abscess. With diffusion of the
infection, pain increases, a high fever of 103° - 104° may occur,
there is severe malaise and marked cervical lymphadenitis. Pus
forming within the marrow spaces of the bone may ooze from the
gingival margins of the teeth which may become very mobile. Overlying soft tissues become swollen and trismus may occur. Involvement of the inferior dental canal may cause anaesthesia of the
mental area. There is a marked leukocytosis. Diagnosis is
entirely from this clinical picture, there being no characteristic
radiographic changes at this stage of the condition before
redistribution of the calcified tissues has taken place.

A similar, but much restricted, inflammatory process occurs in
the case of an infected tooth socket. A distribution of nomenclature is often made to describe this localized condition as an
osteitis, although there is no real pathological difference between it and the more active form.

Following inadequate treatment or partial resolution a chronic
phase may occur in which the leading symptoms are the sequestrat-
ion of fragments of bone which have lost their source of nutrition
together with repair attempts which take the form of calcification immediately below the periosteal layer. The formation of an
involucrum - a complete cuff of newly calcified tissue outside
the normal bone contour - is not usual, but some reparative
attempt on the part of the periosteum is usual. The degree of
bone loss may be considerable and pathological fracture may occur.
The classic description of the radiographic appearance of the
bone at this stage is "moth-eaten" which describes well the
rather blurred and ragged outlines of the bone. Chronic sinuses
discharging pus are a feature of this stage of the disease which
may be protracted over a considerable period with occasional

117

acute exacerbations.

   Acute infantile osteomyelitis, in contradistinction to the
adult form, occurs typically in the maxilla and usually as the
result of a blood-borne infection, although localized trauma may
occasionally provide a route of infection. In this infantile
form staph. aureus is usually the organism involved. The condition occurs predominantly in very young children - under the age
of one year. The leading symptoms are cellulitis of the overlying soft tissues, fever reaching 103° - 104°, evident toxaemia
and a marked leukocytosis. Pus may be discharged from oral or
facial sinuses. Diagnosis is by the clinical signs which, in
view of the dramatic onset and rapid development, are almost
unmistakable.

   A localized form of chronic osteomyelitis occurs with low-
grade infections of long standing in which the characteristic
change is of osteosclerosis. This is variously described as
condensing osteitis, sclerosing osteitis and chronic sclerosing
osteomyelitis. The condition may be localized, in which case
the clinical symptoms are minor - often being confined to an
inflammatory reaction in the overlying mucosa - or absent altog-
ether. The differential diagnosis between such an area of
sclerotic bone and an exostosed retained root is difficult,
although the absence of any detectable root canal or periodontal
membrane gives significant evidence in favour of sclerotic bone.

Dystrophic Bone Lesions
   Only two lesions of this type are seen with any degree of
frequency in the jaws. These are Fibrous dysplasia, which may be
counted as relatively common, and Paget's disease which, although
by no means rare, does not often present primarily as an oral
condition for diagnosis.

   Fibrous dysplasia. This is a term used to describe two somewhat differing conditions. Polystotic fibrous dysplasia
(Albright's disease) is a condition in which multiple areas of
bone are replaced by fibrous tissue containing widely variable
amounts of new ossification. The bony lesions are associated
with skin pigmentation and, in some cases, sexual precocity. In
this condition the active nature of the bone pathology is shown
by a moderate increase in the serum alkaline phosphatase and
calcium levels with no accompanying fall in phosphorus level
(Table XIII).

   Monostotic fibrous dysplasia is a much more common condition
in the jaws. In this disease also there is replacement of the
normal bone architecture by a partially ossified fibrous mass.
This is the only symptom of the disease, there being none of the
hormonal or serum changes shown in polystotic fibrous dysplasia.
The condition occurs in both males and females and the symptoms
are entirely of bone growth. The lesion occurs more often in the
maxilla than in the mandible and in this site may affect the orb-
ital floor and may partially obliterate the antrum (Fig. 7.1).
The radiographic appearance varies according to the extent and
texture of the calcifications within the fibrous tissue, but in

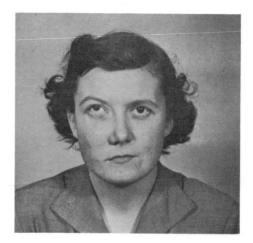

Fig. 7.1. Fibrous dysplasia of the right
maxilla. The facial deformity is evident.

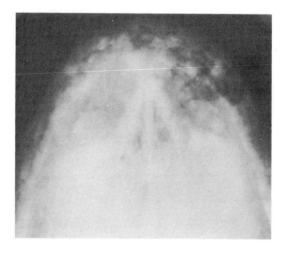

Fig. 7.2. Radiograph of skull in Paget's
disease. This demonstrates the so-called
"cotton wool" appearance of the bone in this
condition.

general presents a mottled appearance, although in a well-
calcified lesion the mottling is minimal. The lesion is confined
to a single bone and is said not to cross suture lines. Differential diagnosis must be made from neoplastic lesions and for
this purpose bone biopsy is necessary. There was in the past
some hesitancy about this procedure in suspected cases of fibrous
dysplasia as malignancy was thought to be caused by the surgical
interference. In fact, however, no case of malignant transformation in non-radiated fibrous dysplasia has ever been reported
and there is no contra-indication at all to biopsy on these
grounds.

   Paget's disease (osteitis deformans). Paget's disease of
bone (to distinguish it from Paget's disease of the nipple - a
form of carcinoma) is a growth disorder of bone which may be
widespread throughout the body but which may show early symptoms
in or about the jaws. It occurs in males and females, usually
over the age of forty and occurs fairly frequently in the maxilla, but very rarely in the mandible. The characteristic of the
condition is the replacement of the normal bone by a pathological
tissue in which bone formation and resorption take place simult-
aneously in a connective tissue mass. The disease occurs in
active and passive phases in which resorption and recalcification
respectively predominate. The end result is of growth and distortion of the bone. The radiographic picture is of a patchy
cotton wool nature which, locally, may simulate other conditions.
Over a wider area, however, the appearance is suggestive if not
absolutely diagnostic (Fig. 7.2). Clinically the earliest complaint may be of an ill-fitting upper denture - although the
classical complaint is of a too small hat. In later stages
obvious deformation may occur and secondary effects such as deafness may accompany closure of the foramina of the base of the
skull. Pain is also a symptom. This may be of two kinds, a
neuralgia-like pain due to compression of nerves at foramina and
a dull 'bone pain' emanating from the affected bone itself. This
latter pain characteristically responds to treatment of the disease with calcitonin. A further point which may help in recognition of the condition is the extreme degree of hypercementosis
which may occur in the teeth standing in an involved area. This
is often clearly seen radiographically. Diagnosis is by full
skeletal radiography and by study of serum chemistry. In Paget's
disease the most striking change in the serum is a great elevat-
ion of the alkaline phosphatase levels (Table XIII). Biopsy may
be carried out, but this is attended by some difficulty since the
new bone growth is often highly vascularized and since the wound
may be slow to heal and liable to infection. On the whole, if
diagnosis may be made by serum and radiographic studies, biopsy
is best avoided.

   Hyperparathyroidism. Although hyperparathyroidism is evidently not primarily a bony condition it produces secondary
effects on the calcified tissues which make it necessary to consider it as a possible diagnosis in some instances of bone lesions. In established hyperparathyroidism there is increased
mobility of the bodily calcium which may lead to calcium withdrawal from the bones. Abnormalities of bone structure produced

TABLE XIII

BLOOD CHEMISTRY IN DISEASES OF BONE

	Ca	p	Alk. Phos.
Normal (conventional units)	8.5 - 11.5	2.5 - 5.0	variable (see below)
Normal (S.I. units)	2.2 - 2.7	0.8 - 1.4	
Paget's disease	N	N	++
Monostotic Fibrous dysplasia	N	N	N
Polystotic Fibrous dysplasia	+	N	+
Hyperparathyroidism	+	-	+

Serum levels of calcium, phosphorus and alkaline phosphatase.

Ca and P in mg/100 ml. (conventional), m.mol/l (S.I.)

Alkaline phosphatase values - normal levels for the age group should be determined from the specific laboratory. Usual adult values up to 375 I.U.

N represents normal

+ represents a moderate rise

++ represents a marked rise

- represents a moderate fall

as a result of this calcium withdrawal are of several kinds but
those in the area of the jaws typically take the form of central
giant cell lesions or giant cell epulides. It is therefore necessary to carry out blood chemistry studies on patients with
either of these lesions. An increase in serum calcium is the
most sensitive early indicator of hyperparathyroidism and if this
is detected in a patient with a giant cell lesion, either central
or peripheral, then suspicions should be aroused and the patient
referred for further assessment.

Cysts
    There are almost as many classifications of the cysts of the
jaws as authors who have written about them. These classifications depend on a consideration both of the morphology of the
cyst in relation to the associated dental structures and also to
the tissue of origin. For instance odontogenic cysts may be
classified as apical or dentigerous when related to teeth or as
primordial when the cyst replaces a tooth. It has recently
become quite evident that an even more important differentiation
depends on the nature of the epithelium lining the cyst. It is a
matter of clinical and histological observation that those odontogenic cysts in which the epithelial lining shows keratinization
are highly susceptible to recurrence whereas those with non-
keratinizing linings rarely do so (except as a result of inadequate surgery). So far as odontogenic cysts are concerned the
differentiation between keratinizing and non-keratinizing
(keratocysts) is of great significance.

    Apart from cysts of odontogenic origin it is necessary to
consider other cysts which occasionally occur in the jaws. Table
XIV lists the cysts considered here.

    Odontogenic keratocysts. It is important that these cysts
should be recognised because of their tendency to recur after
treatment as normally applied to odontogenic cysts. This tendency may be at least partially due to the frequent occurrence of
small daughter cysts in relation to the main cavity, but it is
possible there is some form of intrinsic behaviour which renders
these lesions suceptible to recurrence. It has been suggested
that all primordial cysts and many dentigerous cysts may be of
the keratocyst type although other, apparently periapical cysts
may also be included in this group.

    Initial diagnosis cannot usually be carried out on a clinical
basis although certain features characteristic of the odontogenic keratocyst have been described. It would seem that frequently the growth of the keratocyst is in an anterior-posterior
direction with relatively little lateral expansion of the bone.
It is thus possible for the cyst to attain quite a large size
without it being noticed by the patient. It is common for the
cysts to become secondarily infected and this may well result in
the first symptoms. It has been pointed out that many of the
clinical features of the odontogenic keratocyst may also be
exhibited by an ameloblastoma and this is an important differential diagnosis.

TABLE XIV

CYSTS OF THE JAWS

(1)   ODONTOGENIC ORIGIN
      (may be keratocysts or non keratocysts)

        (a) Periapical (may be subdivided according
            to location)
            Includes residual cysts.

              - mostly non keratocysts

        (b) Dentigerous

              - includes a significant number of
                keratocysts.

        (c) Primordial

              - a high proportion of keratocysts.

(2)   NON ODONTOGENIC ORIGIN

        (a) Developmental (inclusion)

              - epithelial lined

        (b) Haemorrhagic (traumatic, solitary)

              - no lining. Contents - clot, fluid.

        (c) Aneurismal

              - no lining. Contents - blood.

_____

THIS IS A SIMPLIFIED CLASSIFICATION

See text for diagnostic significance
of cyst linings and contents.

Pre-operative assessment of the nature of an odontogenic cyst
depends on aspiration. This simple procedure is sufficient to
distinguish between a cystic lesion, a solid lesion and an air
space as well as providing samples of fluid contents for analysis. The fluid aspirated from a non-keratocyst is generally not
infected and contains glittering crystals of cholesterol. The
fluid aspirated from the keratocyst somewhat resembles pus but in
fact contains desquamated keratinised cells. Histological examination of the aspirated fluid may well give a positive diagnosis.

It has been shown that the level of soluble proteins present
in the cyst fluid is greater than 5.0 grams per 100 millilitres
in non-keratinizing cysts. In odontogenic keratocysts the corresponding protein level is below 4.0 grams per 100 millilitres.
Estimation of the soluble protein content of the cyst fluid is a
further valuable guide to the nature of the cyst.

However, it is true to say that final diagnosis of a keratocyst must be made on histological examination of the tissue
following operation. Biopsy of a cystic lesion before the definitive operation is notoriously prone to lead to problems with
secondary infection and delayed healing and the aspiration methods outlined above are therefore particularly useful in pre-
operative assessment of these lesions.

Periapical cyst (radicular cyst). The most common cystic lesions within the jaw bones are dental cysts associated with inflammatory change about the apices of non-vital teeth. The
originating tooth may be present or may have been extracted
leaving the residual cyst behind. The clinical features shown
by a cyst depend largely on its size. The gradual transformation
from precystic apical granuloma to cyst and its subsequent expansion is a completely painless process unless secondary infection
intervenes, and the cyst may attain a very large size whilst
giving no trouble of any kind to the patient. Under these circumstances the clinical features may be restricted to the expansion of the bone by the cyst and the consequent increase in deformity. Such expansion normally occurs to very much the major
extent on the buccal or labial aspects of the maxilla or mandible. Lingual or palatal expansion is rarely so marked. The
texture of the expanded area depends on the degree of active bone
resorption taking place. If there is a thin wall of relatively
mature bone present, then the classical eggshell cracking of this
may occur on pressure. More often, however, the thin wall overlying the cyst consists of bone undergoing active growth change
and the texture is much softer and rubbery, reflecting the large
proportion of connective tissue present in the bone wall. The
fluid content of the cyst produces a resilient effect on
pressure, although a true fluid thrill cannot be felt in the
partially bone enclosed cavity. A non-vital tooth or teeth may
be present and there may be some mobility of teeth involved
apically in the cyst or displaced by it. Radiographic examination shows a single radiolucent area which may or may not be
associated with a tooth root and which is classically distinguished by a radiopaque line about its periphery (Fig. 7.3). If

the expansion of the cyst has been relatively free and unencumb-
ered then the shape is roughly spherical, but this is much modified by local anatomy. The radiopaque periphery of the cyst is
not a constant feature and, when secondary infection has
occurred, it is often completely absent. Diagnosis of a cyst can
never be made with certainty from radiographic evidence alone.
Confirmation of the nature of the lesion is carried out by aspiration biopsy pre-operatively whilst the non-keratinizing nature
of the epithelial lining is confirmed by histological study
following surgery.

Dentigerous cyst Dentigerous cysts, arising from the foll-
icles of unerupted teeth, rarely grow to a great size and are
often discovered on radiographic examination to establish the
presence of missing teeth (Fig. 7.4). A greater degree of expansion occurs when the unerupted tooth is left behind following
extraction of other teeth and, in these circumstances, bone
expansion may become obvious. Occasionally, particularly in the
maxilla, the dentigerous cyst may grow to a considerable size and
may displace the originating tooth widely. Usually, however, the
bone deformity is not so great as might be expected, the expansion taking place within the normal size and shape of the bone.

Radiographically the dentigerous cyst appears as a radiolucent
area associated with the crown of the responsible tooth. The
shape of the cyst varies widely since it may be greatly modified
by the presence of the roots of adjacent standing teeth, but when
unconstricted it tends to assume a spherical shape. Whatever the
size or shape of the cyst it is generally seen to be enclosing
the crown of the tooth and to be attached to it along a line
approximating to the amelo-cemental junction. The cyst grows
coronally away from the tooth and does not usually grow apically
to include the tooth root. This position of the cyst in relation
to the tooth is highly diagnostic and is retained even if the
tooth is displaced by cyst growth. Only when secondary infection
destroys the normal arrangement of tissues does an appreciable
amount of root surface become included in the cyst cavity. The
margin of a dentigerous cyst does not in general show the radiographically clearly marked line of hypercalcification often
present in the dental cyst.

Initial diagnosis is by the clinical picture and by the radiographic appearance. Aspiration biopsy of the cyst contents may
be made to confirm the nature of the lesion and the tissue removed at surgery should be submitted for histological examination.
A proportion of dentigerous cysts are found to be keratocysts.

Primordial cyst. This term is used to describe a cyst which
has developed from the primitive dental tissues, either in place
of a tooth or as an extension of the dental lamina. There are,
therefore, two possible sites for these cysts.

    1. Replacing a missing tooth.
    2. Between the standing teeth or distal to the third
        molars.

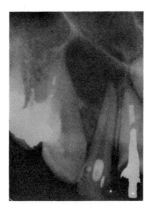 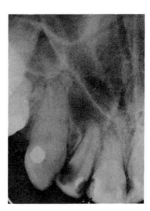

Fig. 7.3. The two periapical radiographs demonstrate the classical appearance of a small periapical cyst. That on the right shows a more clearly defined radio opaque line about its periphery.

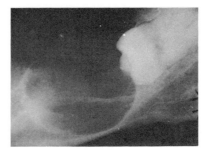

Fig. 7.4. Dentigerous cyst associated with an unerupted mandibular molar. Almost the full thickness of bone has been lost.

Radiographically these cysts may appear to be single or multilocular. An important diagnostic point is that they may be
apparently associated with otherwise quite normal and vital teeth
which may be displaced by the cyst. A high proportion of primordial cysts are keratocysts and in the absence of evidence to the
contrary they should be considered to be of this type unless
proved otherwise. The diagnosis of keratocysts is discussed
above.

Developmental cyst (inclusion cyst) Developmental bone cysts
derived from epithelial remnants included during fusion of embryonic processes may occur on any of the sutural lines, real or
embryonic, in the maxilla or mandible. The usual sites are in the
midline of the palate, the incisive canal and the line of fusion
of maxilla and premaxilla (globulomaxillary cyst). In general
these cysts do not grow to a large size and are symptomless
unless secondary infection occurs. If unobstructed the cysts are
spherical in form and appear on radiography as radiolucent areas,
generally without any well-defined radiopaque margin. These cysts
are not associated with a non-vital tooth and tend to cause
slight separation of the teeth encountered during expansion
rather than erosion of the apices. Teeth of which the apices
appear on radiographs to be in close contact with such a cyst do
not lose their neurovascular supply and remain clinically vital.
This is the important differential point when considering the
possibility of a dental cyst.

Absolute diagnosis is only by examination of a surgical specimen to show non-odontogenic epithelium within the lining, but
since surgical intervention may not be contemplated in a quiescent lesion, differential diagnosis from a solid osteolytic
lesion may be made by aspiration biopsy of the fluid cyst contents.

Haemorrhagic cyst (traumatic cyst, solitary bone cyst) Considerable diagnostic difficulty may be caused by this rare, but
well-recognized lesion, which is apparently a self-healing lesion
of the mandible brought about by trauma in the young patient. It
presents as a simple unlined cavity in the bone which may involve
the apices of several teeth. The edges of the lesion appear
radiographically diffuse and without a well-marked margin. The
lesion is seen in patients of the ten to twenty years of age
group and predominantly in males. Clinical symptoms may include
painless swelling of the bone and, very occasionally, parasthesia
of the inferior dental nerve. Teeth involved remain vital. There
is no change in the blood calcium, phosphorus or alkaline phosphatase. Aspiration produces either a clear yellow fluid or
altered blood and clot. Final diagnosis is by surgical exploration when it is found that the lesion simply consists of an
unlined hole in the bone. This lesion must be distinguished from
the extremely rare "latent bone cyst" (Stafne's bone cavity) of
the mandible which consists of an inclusion of salivary gland
tissue in the lower border of the angle of the mandible. This
lesion lies invariably below and behind the inferior dental canal
and is a static developmental abnormality. Aspiration shows the

contents to be non-fluid whilst surgical or sialographic examination shows the contents to be an extension of normal submandibular salivary gland tissue.

   Aneurysmal bone cyst The aneurysmal bone cyst is a relatively
uncommon lesion which may occur at sites throughout the skeleton
and in the jaws. The patients are usually young. The lesion is
probably essentially vascular although its precise aetiology is
by no means certain. The important diagnostic point, however,
is that it contains blood filled spaces (in a matrix of connective tissue with immature bone and giant cells) and therefore has
a tendency towards profuse haemorrhage on any form of surgical
intervention. This tendency, however, is not so great as in a
haemangioma in which the blood supply is often via large arterial
vessels.

   On x-ray the aneurysmal bone cyst may appear as a single
osteolytic lesion or it may have a multilocular appearance described as being like soap bubbles. In an advanced lesion the
bone of the jaws may be considerably expanded. However, a thin
intact cortical layer is usually seen on the outer surface of
the cyst.

   It should be pointed out that the aneurysmal bone cyst and
the haemorrhagic bone cyst are not epithelial-lined structures
as are the odontogenic cysts. Diagnosis by the histological
appearances of their contents may present some difficulty.

Neoplastic Lesions in Bone
   There is a wide range of possible neoplastic growth within
the bone of the jaws, both primary and secondary. Initial symptoms may be of bone expansion, tooth mobility, inferior dental
nerve anaesthesia or pain. The earliest sign may, however, be
the unexplained appearance of a dental radiograph taken for some
routine diagnostic purpose. Whatever the leading symptoms the
first diagnostic step is likely to be the taking of a radiograph
of the area. The signs which should arouse suspicion include
the presence of an osteolytic area in the bone, a multilocular appearance, erosion of tooth roots, expansion of normal
bone outlines, erosion of cortical plate bone, evidence of new
bone formation in osteolytic areas or gross distortion of normal
bone architecture. If suspicions are thus aroused it is essential to gain as much radiographic information as to the nature
and extent of the lesion as possible (Fig. 7.5).

   Radiographic examination will show with some degree of accuracy the extent of a neoplastic lesion but is not sufficient to
give any more than a tentative diagnosis of the nature of the
lesion. Although typical radiographic appearances are described
for many neoplasms these are in no cases invariable and are
never absolutely diagnostic. This may be due to primary variation from the "normal" in the behaviour of the lesion, to the
presence of infection or unusual localized reaction to the neoplastic process. In some cases the spectrum of neoplastic
tissue produced in various examples of the same basic neoplastic

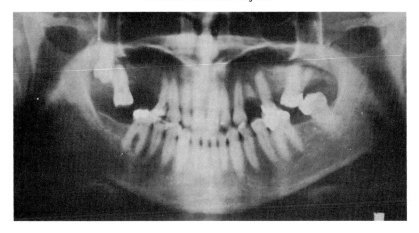

Fig. 7.5 (a)

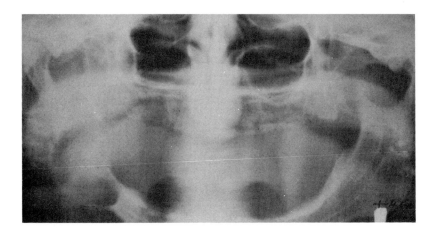

Fig. 7.5 (b)

Fig. 7.5(a). The lesion at the right angle of
the mandible is a secondary carcinoma of the
thyroid. Compare this with the radiograph of a
residual cyst at the same site shown in 7.5 (b).
Although there is some diffuseness of outline the
cyst is generally better delineated than is the
neoplasm. However, diagnosis on x-ray evidence
alone is very uncertain.

process may be in itself sufficient to explain widely differing
radiographic appearances.

Following the observation of a suspicious lesion and if the
diagnostic criteria for simple cystic lesions are not satisfied
then, prior to surgical investigation, blood chemistry studies
must be carried out.   In cases of polystotic fibrous dysplasia,
hyperparathyroidism and multiple myeloma there are changes of
diagnostic significance in the serum calcium, phosphorus and
alkaline phosphatase levels.   Should one of these more generalized conditions be suspected, skeletal radiographs should be
taken in the search for further lesions.   Following such studies
surgical exploration is essential to obtain tissue for the histological examination which is the only absolute diagnostic test.
Incisional biopsy of a central bone neoplasm may be productive of
considerable haemorrhage and suitable facilities should be available to deal with this.   In particular, the incision of a central
haemangioma may be followed by quite uncontrollable and fatal
haemorrhage.   It is strongly suggested that surgical exploration
of any central bone lesion should at all times be preceded by
aspiration to eliminate the possibility of a haemangioma.   Should
this rare lesion be suspected, diagnosis is by local angiography
and incisional biopsy must never be attempted (Chapter 1, Figs.
1.3, 1.4).

Chapter VIII

The Temporomandibular Joint

In considering the diagnosis of symptoms arising from the temporomandibular joint it should be kept in mind that there are two distinct sources of such symptoms. The first arises from the muscles, joint structures and other associated tissues as a result of abnormal physical activity within the joint. The second is from pathological changes in the joint itself. In the first case, there are no primary physical signs within the joint and diagnosis must be made from the history, secondary signs, and symptoms. Abnormalities of movement and function may be of vital importance in giving the diagnosis in these circumstances. In the second of these cases there may be primary physical signs present in the joint to account for the symptoms:- in such circumstances the joint damage may be associated with systemic abnormality - rheumatoid arthritis is an example of this situation.

Differentiation between these two groups of conditions may initially be very difficult. However, it is true that the very large majority of cases of pain and other symptoms arising from the temporomandibular joint do so as a result of a dysfunction syndrome rather than as a result of any primary pathology.

<u>Symptoms in Joint Disorders</u>

1. <u>Pain</u>. The predominant complaint is of pain. This may be felt as a dull ache over the area of the joint, the ear, over the temporal fossa or over the maxilla. The pain may be bilateral or unilateral and is usually described as being constant, but with acute exacerbations. It is during these acute exacerbations that the radiation of the pain from the joint often occurs. In some instances associated pain in the neck, upper arm, occipital area or along the lingual nerve may be reported. The severe attacks of pain occur predominantly in the early morning in some patients, whereas in other patients they are more common at the end of the day. Acute episodes may also be precipitated after a meal, at the wide opening of the mouth, or during the night when lying heavily on one side of the face.

2. <u>Joint sounds</u>. The patient most commonly complains of a click, representing the movement of one component of the joint over the others. This click may be quite loud and readily audible. In other

cases, however, the stethoscope must be used to
hear the sound. Although an acute episode of
pain may be precipitated by the action which
also produces a click, patients find that pain
is usually associated with periods in which
clicking is minimal. Apart from the single
loud click, crepitation-like sounds may be heard
in the joint on stethoscopic examination. Care
must be taken in the use of the stethoscope to
eliminate the crackling sound produced by laying
the bell of the instrument over hair - the
resulting crackling sound can easily be mistaken
for joint crepitation.

3.   Restriction in opening The patient may report
     difficulty in wide opening, often associated with
     the imminent onset of a loud click. In other
     instances the difficulty may be in applying pressure
     on closing the mouth.

4.   Swelling For some not very clear reason, some
     patients with temporomandibular joint disturbances
     complain of swelling over the maxilla. A slight
     degree of soft tissue swelling may be occasionally
     noted in this site on examination. In a few other
     instances patients may complain of tenderness and
     swelling in the area of the parotid - presumably
     an effect brought about by the close proximity of
     part of this gland to the temporomandibular joint.
     In these cases it may be a matter of some difficulty
     to distinguish between parotid involvement in joint
     disturbance or joint involvement in a parotid
     pathology.

Examination of the Joint
     Examination of the temporomandibular joint and face should
begin by observing the degree of symmetry of the mandible and
face and by observing the path of excursion of the mandible on
opening and closing. Loud joint sounds may be heard at this
time. In order to examine the joint by palpation the examiner
should be in front of the patient so that movement of the mandible may be related to those palpated in the condylar heads. A
single finger is placed over each condyle head whilst the mandibular movements are carried out. Abnormal tenderness associated
with the joints is detected by light pressure over the fossa when
the mouth is fully open. Faint joint sounds may be heard by
using a stethoscope placed over the condyle head whilst mandibular movements are performed.

     Following the extra-oral examination a careful note must be
made of the occlusal relationship of the teeth, paying particular
attention to missing teeth, the presence of faceting or any
evidence of bruxism.

     By far the most important abnormality of this kind in the
present context is the absence of molar or premolar teeth,

leading to a lack of posterior tooth support.

Muscular tenderness associated with joint disturbance may be
detected by palpation of the masseters. This is carried out by
asking the patient to clench the teeth firmly together. When
the masseters are thereby put into contraction the examining
finger is run up the anterior border intra-orally, counter
pressure being exerted from the external surface. When the
examining finger reaches the zygomatic origin of the masseter,
tenderness becomes evident and is shown by the patient's reaction.
A similar test should be carried out on the opposite side. This
test for muscular tenderness is a more reliable one than that of
the pterygoid sign. This procedure is misleadingly unpleasant to
the normal patient.

Radiographic techniques used to investigate the joint include
the lateral oblique view, used routinely to demonstrate the anatomy and range of opening of the joint (Fig. 8.1). The condyle
necks and heads are demonstrated well in a high orthopantomograph
view, (Fig. 8.2) although the relation of the condyle heads to
the fossae is not well displayed. Tomography may be used to give
a clear view of the condyle in situ but the clearest view of the
condyle head from the point of view of structural change is given
by the Toller transpharyngeal view (Fig. 8.3). Arthrography, the
injection of the joint spaces with radio-opaque material in order
to delineate joint components, was at one time occasionally advo-
cated for study of the temporomandibular joint but has now been
virtually abandoned as it is difficult and painful and gives rise
to tenderness for some time afterwards.

Electro-myographic studies of the musculature in cases of
temporomandibular joint disturbance show deviations from the
normal pattern of action. This is as yet a research tool but it
is probable that the technique will eventually be valuable as a
diagnostic aid and much work is being carried out to this end.

<u>Chronic temporomandibular joint dysfunction (Pain Dysfunction
Syndrome)</u> This condition is found predominantly (80%) in female
patients. The predominant complaint is of pain, which may take
any of the forms previously described. This pain may be associated with limitation of opening or with joint sounds, also as
previously outlined. The patients quite often admit to a history
of unusual mental stress although overt psychiatric abnormality
is unusual.

There may be a history of previous joint clicking, limitation
of opening, trauma, or recurrent dislocation. Examination may
show one or several of the following: limitation of opening of
the mouth; deviation of the mandible on opening; clicking heard
or felt in the joint; gross malocclusion leading to abnormal
joint movements or minor degrees of malocclusion with abnormal
cuspal guidance of closure; gross occlusal attrition; occlusal
disharmony resulting from the loss of teeth; poorly articulating
dentures or bite closure resulting from lack of posterior teeth
or unsatisfactory dentures; masseteric tenderness.

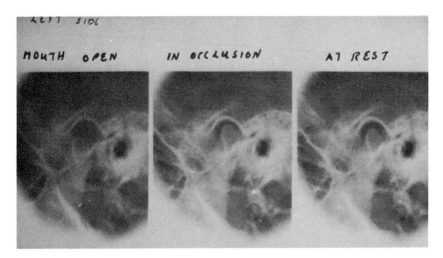

Fig. 8.1. Lateral oblique views of the left
temporo-mandibular joint with the mouth open,
in occlusion and at rest. This is the commonly
used view to demonstrate the relation of the
condyle head to the fossa.

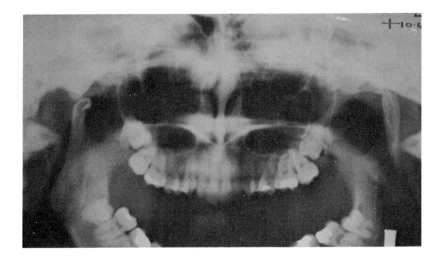

Fig. 8.2. A high orthopantomogram which demonstrates well the morphology of a condyle head
and necks. In this view it will be seen that
there is a difference in morphology between two
condyle heads.

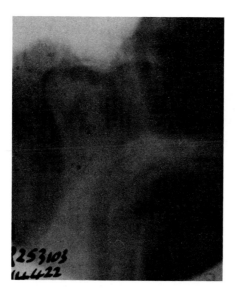

Fig. 8.3. Toller transpharyngeal view of the
condyle head. In this view the x-ray beam is
directed through the coronoid notch from the
opposite side with the mouth wide open. The
beam crosses the pharyngeal space and is unobstructed by bony structures. In this film
rheumatic erosions of the condyle surface are
shown. The Toller view is very useful to show
such pathological changes.

Questioning may reveal the presence of a habit of mandibular positioning or action, usually a protrusion or lateral excursion carried out when engaged on some mental activity. There may be a habit of biting on some foreign body such as a pen or pencil or there may be evidence of bruxism, supplied, in the absence of associated attrition, by some other member of the patient's family.

In most patients with chronic temporomandibular joint symptoms, radiographs of the joints reveal no abnormality of structure although limitation or increase in joint movement may be seen.

Care must be taken in differentiating the pain due to temporomandibular joint disturbances from that arising from dental causes or from facial pain of the types described in Chapter IV. In particular, the differential diagnosis between facial pain of psychogenic origin and that caused by joint dysfunction in patients undergoing mental stress is difficult. In fact, the two conditions occasionally seem to merge in a patient with physical signs of temporomandibular joint dysfunction, but with the demonstrative, anxious, obsessive outlook typical of the patient converting hidden anxieties into facial pain symptoms. Needless to say, in such cases, the first presumptive diagnosis must be of joint dysfunction and only if all physical signs of this have been cleared by treatment must the diagnosis of psychogenic pain be more firmly entertained. It is in observing the reaction to treatment that the differential diagnosis is perhaps best made, all treatment, of whatever kind, failing in the case of the pain of psychogenic origin.

Rheumatoid arthritis. It was previously thought that the temporomandibular joint was rarely involved in cases of generalised rheumatic disease. It has recently been shown, however, that this is not so and that there is evidence of its involvement in two-thirds of all cases of the disease. In an investigation by Ogus, 62 patients with established rheumatoid arthritis were examined, of whom 61% had evidence of involvement of the temporomandibular joint. The major complaint was of pain followed by aching, stiffness and crepitus. On examination, crepitus was found to be the most commonly occurring clinical sign, followed by tenderness of the joint and the existence of a functional abnormality. Radiographic evidence of changes was found in a high proportion of these patients, presenting as erosions, proliferations and flattening of the condylar head. As in other joints, the disease process may occur in a phasic manner, acute exacerbations being followed by either a healing phase or a secondary chronic phase.

Immunological tests for rheumatoid arthritis have been outlined in Chapter II. These tests may prove positive before systemic changes have been noticed.

Osteo-arthritis (Osteoarthrosis). Changes may take place in the temporomandibular joint as part of a generalized arthritic

condition. In this case the history is usually of gradually
increasing stiffness and pain. The joint may be tender to pressure and crepitations may be heard and felt when the joint is
moved. Most patients are female and over the age of 50. The
R.A. factor is negative and the E.S.R. normal in these patients.

Radiographically the joint space is reduced and there may be
some erosions of the articulating surfaces of the condyle and of
the fossa.

Hyperplasia of the condyle. This rare condition, which is
usually unilateral, may be due to the retention, in an active
state, of the condylar growth cartilage after the age at which
it normally becomes quiescent. Alternatively, it may be due to
a pathologically overactive growth centre at the normal age.

There is a history of a slowly progressive lengthening of one
side of the mandible with resultant deviation of the mandible
away from the affected side. The diagnosis may be assisted by
photographs of the patient taken at intervals over the years
during which the condition has occurred and if such a series can
be assembled it seems almost invariably the case that the condition can be seen for some time before it was noticed by the
patient. There is often gross malocclusion produced and pain may
be present due to mechanical factors of pressure and joint dysfunction.

Radiographs show the enclosed condyle head with a uniform
structure not resembling a neoplasm.

Ankylosis. Ankylosis of one or both temporomandibular joints
is rare. It is practically always due to trauma acting on the
area of the joint. This may be direct mechanical trauma or, more
frequently, may be the result of an inflammatory process taking
place in or about the joint. Rheumatoid arthritis, osteomyelitis
and gonorrhoea have been most often recorded as the initiating
factors. If the traumatic process has resulted in complete
ossification of the joint area then true ankylosis is the result.
Partial ossification may occur with the production of a partial
fibrous joint.

In many cases the traumatic process destroys or damages the
condylar growth centre. If this is done before development is
complete the result is failure of forward and downward growth of
the mandible (micrognathia).

Acute dislocation. There is usually a history of some unusually
wide opening of the mouth, such as in biting a large food mass or
in yawning. The dislocation is practically always bilateral. The
mouth is fixed in a wide open position and palpation of the joint
area reveals a depression over the articular fossa, whilst the
condyle head may be felt prominently placed in front of the fossa.
Radiographs confirm the condyle head to be in this anterior position. Backward dislocation occurs only in cases of severe
trauma and is very rare.

Chapter IX

Facial Swellings: Lesions of Salivary Glands

Infections originating in the teeth have been discussed in Chapter V together with some other, less common, infections of non-odontogenic origin with which they may be confused. It must always be remembered that, although dental infections are by far the most common cause of swellings about the face to be seen by the dental surgeon, there are many other possibilities which must be considered in a differential diagnosis.

Allergic reactions. Allergic reactions such as angioneurotic oedema or giant urticaria sometimes occur on the face and are occasionally seen in the tongue and palate. There is localized swelling of the soft tissues, usually preceded and accompanied by irritation and itching. The swelling may appear quickly (in a matter of minutes) and, if untreated, disappears in upwards of 12 hours. There is frequently a history of specific sensitivity and a family history of allergic conditions.

An extensive angioneurotic oedema involving tongue, pharynx, palate and larynx may occur as a response to drugs, especially antibiotics, in an allergic individual. The onset of such a condition shortly following a dose of penicillin or other antibiotic may occur in a previously unsensitized individual, or in one with no history of allergic manifestations. The condition is one of great danger and anyone administering antibiotics must be prepared to recognize it and to apply emergency treatment at once.

Neoplasia. Neoplastic growth within the soft tissues of the face is rare. When it does occur, however, it is vital that a diagnosis should be made quickly. The signs and symptoms are of a swelling, usually growing slowly, generally painless and not tender to pressure. Palpation reveals its solid nature. The diagnosis is entirely by biopsy examination of the tissue. Radiographic examination reveals no abnormality in an early case. If, however, there has been bone infiltration, extreme care must be taken to differentiate between this and inflammatory changes of an odontogenic origin.

Masseteric hypertrophy. Unilateral enlargement of the muscles of mastication, and of the masseter in particular, occasionally occurs as a response to serious derangement of the occlusion leading to unilateral mastication. It may also, however, occur with little or no occlusal disharmony and, in fact, may be bilateral rather than unilateral. In the affected patients the complaint is usually only of increasing facial assymetry. On examination the masseter (or masseters) are found to be enlarged as a whole, often with a marked increase overlying the mandibular insertion. When the masseter is defined for examination by asking the patient to clench the teeth the muscle is easily palpated, the lower part often standing out and resembling a soft tissue mass. On radiography the mandibular insertion of the masseter may be represented by a marked concavity at the periphery of which there is lipping of the bone. If electromyographic facilities are available it is possible to demonstrate atypical muscle activity in all the muscles of mastication.

This is a rather mysterious condition and little is known of its aetiology. Diagnosis is entirely by clinical examination as outlined above.

Enlargement of the Lymph Nodes of the Face and Neck

Examination. Normal lymph nodes are not palpable. Enlargement of a node or a change in texture, so that it may be palpated through the skin, indicates either that the node is taking part in the bodily defence mechanism acting against an infection, or that there is some basic pathological change within the node itself. Differentiation between these two situations is vital.

Lymph nodes may be examined by palpation or by biopsy, usually of the excisional type, although aspiration biopsy may occasionally be used. When examining the lymph nodes of the head and neck each of the main groups must be palpated in turn, whilst the surrounding tissues are relaxed by bending the patient's head forward and laterally towards the side examined. From a position behind the patient the facial, submandibular, submental, parotid, cervical, auricular and occipital groups of nodes are palpated in turn on each side. If a palpable node is found, its texture is noted and it is moved between two fingers to discover any attachment to skin, underlying tissue or adjacent nodes.

Acute infections. Lymphadenitis arising from an acute infection such as a periapical lesion, a parodontal abscess or a pericoronitis is usually unilateral. The appearance of the nodes is rapid, they are soft and are painful when touched. There may be oedema of the soft tissue surrounding the nodes giving the visual impression of greater enlargement than is, in fact, the case. The facial lymph node - lying just anterior to the anterior border of masseter at the level of the occlusal plane - is commonly involved in children and may give rise to difficulty in identification.

Chronic infections. In chronic infections the affected nodes are firm and not tender. They do not become attached to the skin or surrounding tissues and do not coalesce. In long-standing cases of chronic infection, calcification of a node may present as a solitary hard, non-fixed swelling. More widespread smaller calcifications in the cervical nodes are more common. They are usually discovered incidentally during radiography, are asymptomatic and cannot be palpated.

Secondary neoplasia. Spread to lymph nodes of the neck may occur at any stage in the growth of a malignant neoplasm of the

oral cavity, pharynx, antrum or related structures. The nodes
are initially painless, hard and usually unilateral. In the
early stages the enlarged lymph nodes may show only non specific
inflammatory changes on biopsy. In later stages the nodes may
become painful because of secondary infection, may coalesce, or
may become fixed to the skin or surrounding tissues. Diagnosis
is confirmed by excision biopsy of the nodes.

Leukaemia. In all types of leukaemia generalized lymph node
enlargement may be an early symptom. The nodes are at first
usually discrete and painless but may grow to a very large size.
This response is very variable, even within a specific type of
leukaemia. Diagnosis is by blood examination and marrow biopsy.

Hodgkin's disease. The early signs of Hodgkin's disease may
be a swelling of the lymph nodes of the neck. The nodes are
discrete and painless and have the consistency of rubber. Early
in the course of the disease there is often a secondary anaemia
together with a leucocytosis and a monocytosis which may be up to
15 per cent. These changes are, however, non specific and firm
diagnosis is made by biopsy of an affected node.

Microscopic examination shows the normal structure of the node
to be replaced by a tissue including specific multinucleated
cells known as Reed Steinberg cells.

Infective monomucleosis (glandular fever). Cervical lymphadenitis is an important sign of this viral disease. The nodes are
moderately enlarged, discrete and tender to pressure. There is a
febrile reaction, sometimes with rigors, a sore throat and there
are occasionally petachiae on the palate. Blood examination
shows a leukocytosis, largely due to the presence of specific
cells, known as Downey cells, which are in appearance midway
between a lymphocyte and a monocyte. The Paul-Bunnell test is
the specific antibody reaction for this condition, although the
Wassermann reaction may also be positive (see Chapter III).

Lesions of the Major Salivary Glands
Only two basic techniques are widely used for the investigation of salivary gland disease. These are, firstly, careful
clinical examination and, secondly, radiography - including the
use of contrast media. Biopsy study of minor salivary gland
tissue from the lip is also a convenient method of indirectly
obtaining information about the salivary tissue in general and
avoids the difficult and somewhat hazardous process of a biopsy
of a major gland. In specialist centres facilities may be available for carrying out of salivary flow rate determinations and
radio-isotope tracer studies of gland function.

Clinical examination. The parotid gland, lying as it does
partially concealed by the ascending ramus of the mandible, is
not easy to palpate. Tenderness and swelling is best detected by
standing in front of the patient and by placing the fingers over
the posterior border of the ascending ramus of the mandible.
Backwards and inwards movement of the fingers with light pressure
is almost always sufficient to detect tenderness in the super-

ficial part of the parotid.   This manoeuvre is necessary to
differentiate parotid tenderness from that of the masseter or
temporomandibular joint with which it is often confused.   When
examining a parotid gland care must be taken to also examine the
duct papilla for signs of inflammatory change.   The saliva can be
best assessed for a purulent content or some similar abnormality
by lightly compressing the skin overlying the area of the duct
with the fingers.   If the cheek is held retracted the saliva
expressed by this manoeuvre will be seen coursing downwards from
the duct over the buccal mucosa.   Subjective assessments of flow
rate of saliva made in this way are, however, completely unreli-
able.

The submandibular gland is palpated below the angle and body
of the mandible, this simple palpation being reinforced by bimanual palpation with a finger in the floor of the mouth, gentle
pressure being exerted between the examining hands and finger. As
in the case of the parotid gland the duct should be observed for
signs of inflammation and a subjective assessment made of the
quality of the saliva.   The sublingual glands may be palpated in
the same manner and using a similar technique.

Sialography.   Sialography is carried out by injecting into the
duct of the appropriate gland a radio opaque fluid.   Immediately
after injection radiographs of the area are taken and, if the
technique has been satisfactory, a well outlined image of the
secretory and duct system of the gland is given.

The material most often used for the injection is an iodized
poppy seed oil which owes its radio opacity to its high iodine
content (40 per cent).   Approximately 3 ml of the fluid are
injected into the duct papilla using a needle of 18 to 14 gauge.
As soon as the injection is completed the desired radiographs are
taken.   An abnormal sialogram is shown in Fig. 9.2.   In the most
recent techniques water soluble media of satisfactory properties
have been introduced and the injection is made by hydrostatic
pressure - this gives more reproducible results than the use of
syringes.

Calculi.   Calculus formation is most common in the submandibular gland, next, but not nearly so commonly, in the parotid
gland and rarely in the sublingual gland.   The calculi often come
to notice only when an attempt is made to expel them through the
duct.   Impaction may occur and symptoms then arise.   In the case
of the parotid, calculus impaction is likely to occur at the
point where the duct makes a sharp turn to pierce the buccinator
muscle.   This is at the anterior margin of the masseter muscle.
In the submandibular duct there are two major points of impaction.
The first is as the duct bends over the posterior free edge of
mylohyoid.   The second and most frequent point for impaction is
at a constriction just before the duct opens into the floor of
the mouth at its papilla.   At this point a calculus can be often
palpated through the thin overlying tissues (Fig. 9.1).

The symptoms of salivary calculus are due to obstruction of

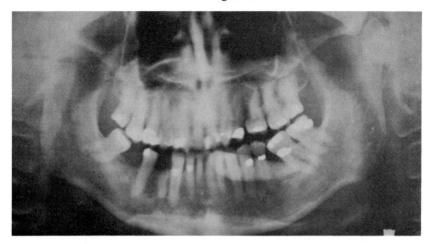

Fig. 9.1. A very large submandibular calculus
is shown superimposed on the teeth of the left
mandible. A calculus of this size, impacted in
the submandibular duct, is palpable through the
floor of the mouth

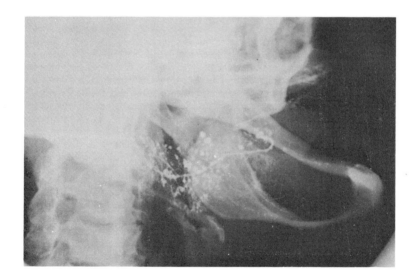

Fig. 9.2. Sialogram of parotid gland showing
terminal dilatation of the ducts.

the salivary flow. Swelling of the gland with a sensation of
pressure followed by pain localized in the gland typically
appears at meal times, or whenever the salivary flow is stimulated. After the meal the pain subsides and the swelling slowly
reduces. In long standing cases there is frequently some permanent degree of swelling of the gland. The symptoms are easily
reproduced during examination by stimulating the salivary flow
by a piece of lemon or some other sialogogue.

Diagnosis is made by the history and by the reproduction of
symptoms on salivary stimulation. The calculus may well be
palpable within the duct. In the case of the submandibular duct
bimanual palpation should be used, one hand being used to lift
the floor of the mouth. When palpating for calculi great care
must be taken not to force the calculus back towards the gland
since a peripherally placed calculus is simple to remove, but a
centrally placed one difficult. For this reason probing of the
duct should never be carried out simply to confirm the presence
of a calculus. Very occasionally a submandibular calculus may
ulcerate through the overlying tissue and present as an ulcer
with, apparently, a hard base.

Clinical findings are confirmed by radiography. A calculus is
almost always seen on an occlusal film for the submandibular and
sublingual glands, and on a lateral oblique film for the parotid
gland. Occasionally, however, a poorly calcified calculus may
not show up on radiography, and sialography may be necessary to
demonstrate the site of obstruction.

Acute infections. Most acute bacterial infections of the
salivary glands are secondary to obstruction. In past years
ascending parotitis was a frequent and serious complication of
abdominal surgery, but with the advent of antibiotics the incidence of this has been greatly reduced.

Diagnosis is by the history of pain and swelling and by the
evidence of purulent saliva discharging from an inflamed duct
and papilla. This secondary inflammation of the duct is almost
invariable and is an important diagnostic point. Trismus is
often present in an acute parotitis, and the pressure may initiate the auriculotemporal syndrome (Chapter IV). Radiography
will show little and sialography is hardly possible and might
indeed be dangerous in an acute infection.

Chronic infections. Chronic infection may be the result of
inadequate treatment of an acute condition, or may arise by a
direct chronic process, particularly when calculi are involved.

The symptoms are of long-standing discomfort in the gland,
together with some permanent swelling. There are frequently
acute exacerbations. The saliva discharging from the duct is
scanty and purulent. The ducts often undergo fibrosis and
constriction with terminal dilatation within the substance of
the gland. Sialography is valuable to confirm the diagnosis
(Fig. 9.2).

Mumps. Mumps (epidemic parotitis) is an infection of the
parotid glands (and, occasionally, submandibular glands) by a
specific virus and there may be a history of contact with a previous case (incubation period 2 to 3 weeks). It may be unilateral, but is usually to some extent bilateral.

The symptoms are of malaise, fever, nausea and abdominal
pains. These are succeeded by swelling of the gland or glands,
giving rise to considerable pain and tenderness to pressure.
Characteristic is the filling up of the space behind the mandible and below the ear by the swollen gland. Opening of the
mouth causes pressure on the swollen gland and is painful. There
may be some inflammation of the duct of the affected gland. The
symptoms normally subside after approximately one week although
occasionally complications such as orchitis occur.

Neoplasia. Salivary tumours are relatively common in the parotid gland, less so in the submandibular and sublingual glands.
The neoplasms which arise have a wide range of structure ranging
from simple adenoma-like form, through the bizarre pleomorphic
types of the so-called mixed tumours to the malignant cylindroma
(adenocystic carcinoma). There may also be frank squamous carcinoma, sarcoma arising from the connective tissue elements of the
gland and a variety of other neoplasms.

The early clinical findings of all these neoplasms are similar
however. Painless swelling is the predominant symptom, often of
many years duration. In the case of the more benign lesions this
swelling may become enormous before any other symptoms supervene.
Late symptoms are due to pressure by the neoplasm on nearby
structures or by invasion of them. In the case of the parotid
neoplasms this may include the auriculotemporal syndrome, or
rarely, a facial nerve paralysis. In the case of the cylindroma,
silent metastases may be present early in the progress of the
disease, particularly in the lungs, and therefore a chest film
should be part of the first investigation.

Differentiation of the neoplasms is by biopsy only, usually
excision biopsy. An accurate assessment of the prognosis of
these lesions in all but the most obviously malignant cases is
difficult, but it is important that careful histological studies
be made to identify the type of the neoplasm. In the case of an
early lesion, sialography may be invaluable in outlining the non-
secreting area of tumour tissue within the gland.

Dry mouth (xerostomia). Investigation of this troublesome
condition may be difficult. A simple clinical assessment of the
flow of saliva is likely to be extremely inaccurate, and only
after relatively complex investigations can it be determined
whether or not in fact a reduction in salivary flow is present.
In the investigation of the patient complaining of a dry mouth
the initial history taking is of particular importance since a
reduction in salivary flow may accompany certain generalised
auto-immune processes, the taking of drugs or may simply be a
consequence of old age. A large number of drugs have been implicated in the production of a dry mouth - perhaps the most common

of these being antihistamines, antihypertensives and psycho-
tropic drugs.

If a relatively simple explanation for the apparent dryness
is not found on initial examination it may be difficult to determine whether or not further investigation is justifiable. There
is little to be gained from carrying out less than the full
range of investigations as outlined below for the study of
Sjögren's syndrome but in many cases such a full investigation
is not justifiable.

Sjögren's syndrome.   This syndrome consists of three major
components:-

    1. Loss of salivary secreting units.
    2. Loss of lachrymal secretion.
    3. Associated auto-immune disease.

It occurs predominantly in middle-aged female patients and may
also occur in a limited form, without the presence of other auto-
immune disease. In this case it is known as the Sicca syndrome.

The common first complaint of the patient is of a dry mouth
associated with soreness of the oral mucosa. On examination the
patient is seen to have an evidently atrophic mucosa, particularly of the tongue. Conjunctival irritation may occur early or
later in the condition.

The complete investigation of this group of conditions has
been described by Mason & Chisholm as follows:-

    1. Clinical examination of the patient.

    2. Salivary flow estimation. This must
        be done by cannulation, the use of
        collecting cups or some similar device -
        whole saliva samples have been found to
        be unsatisfactory for diagnostic purposes.
        A single representative gland (usually
        the parotid) is chosen for study.

    3. Sialography of a representative gland -
        also usually the parotid.

    4. Labial gland biopsy. In this technique
        a small elipse of tissue is taken from
        the mucosa of the lower lip, together
        with the underlying minor salivary glands.
        The degree of histological change in the
        mucous glands has been shown to be
        directly related to that in the major
        salivary glands. At the same time an
        assessment can be made of the overlying
        mucosal changes.

5. Laboratory studies are carried out for
    the presence of auto-antibodies and, in
    particular, of the R.A. factor.

6. Opthalmic examination should be carried
    out if this is thought necessary.
    Estimation of the rate of tear formation
    may be carried out by absorbing the
    secretion on a folded piece of filter
    paper, but this is considered a relatively
    unreliable test.

7. In some centres where facilities are
    available scintiscanning of the major
    glands may be carried out using radio-
    isotopes. The amount of uptake of the
    isotope is directly proportionate to
    the rate of secretion of the salivary
    glands and the uptake is therefore an
    accurate reflection of secretory
    capacity.

It is evident that a full investigation of the kind outlined
above is a lengthy and complicated matter and not to be undertaken lightly.

Additional Reading

Although the chapters in the present book are relatively
self-contained it is anticipated that they will be read by
the undergraduate in conjunction with the course text books
dealing with the various dental specialities. Clinical
descriptions and illustrations of a wide range of lesions
in and around the mouth are given in the following books:-

A COLOUR ATLAS OF ORAL MEDICINE
Tyldesley, W.R.
Wolfe, London 1978.

A COLOUR ATLAS OF ORO-FACIAL DISEASES
Kay, L.W. & Haskill, R.
Wolfe, London 1971.

SYNDROMES OF THE HEAD AND NECK. 2nd ED.
Gorlin, R.J., Pindborg, J.J. & Cohen, M.M.
McGraw-Hill, New York 1976.

PATHOLOGY OF THE DENTAL HARD TISSUES
Pindborg, J.J.
Munsgaard, Copenhagen 1970.

BENIGN CYSTIC LESIONS OF THE JAWS, THEIR
DIAGNOSIS AND TREATMENT.
Killey, H.C., Kay, L.W. and Seward, G.R.
Churchill Livingstone,
Edinburgh, London and New York 1977.

SALIVARY GLANDS IN HEALTH AND DISEASE
Mason, D.K. and Chisholm, D.M.
W.B. Saunders, London 1975.

TOOTHACHE AND OROFACIAL PAIN. 2nd ED.
Mumford, J.M.
Churchill Livingstone,
Edinburgh, London and New York 1976.

WOLFF'S 'HEADACHE AND OTHER HEAD PAIN' 3rd ED.
Dalessio, D.J. (Ed.)
Oxford University Press, New York 1972.

A great deal of relevant information may also be found in:-

    TEXTBOOK OF DERMATOLOGY. 2nd ED.
Rooke, A.J., Wilkinson, D.S. and Ebling, F.J.G.
Blackwell, Oxford 1973.

    BLOOD AND ITS DISORDERS
Hardisty, R.M. & Weatherall, D.J. (Eds.)
Blackwell Scientific, Oxford 1974.

If further details of laboratory procedures are needed the following books will be found helpful:-

    MEDICAL MICROBIOLOGY
Ed. Cruickshank, R.   12th Edition
Churchill Livingstone, Edinburgh 1973.

    CLINICAL DIAGNOSIS BY LABORATORY METHODS
Todd-Sanford.
Davidson, I. and Henry, J.B. (Eds.)
W.B. Saunders, Philadelphia 1974.

    METABOLIC DISORDERS OF BONE
Patterson, C.R.
Blackwell Scientific, Oxford 1974.

    HANDBOOK OF EXPERIMENTAL IMMUNOLOGY.   2nd ED.
Weir, D.M. (Ed.)
Blackwell Scientific, Oxford 1973.

Index